Dr. T's Drop the Fat Diet

Dr. T's Drop the Fat Diet

12 Steps to a Leaner You Forever

Author Francisco M. Torres, MD, ABPMR

Contributor Gabriel Torres, CSCS

Editor Abby Campbell, BSc, SFN, SSN, CPT

Dr. T's Drop the Fat Diet: 12 Steps to a Leaner You Forever

ISBN-13: 978-0-692-51680-5

1. Health   2. Nutrition

Library of Congress Control Number: 2015950069

Version 1:1

First Printing September 30, 2015

(paperback edition, 7" x 10")

Author: Francisco M. Torres, MD, ABPMR

Contributor: Gabriel Torres, CSCS

Editor: Abby Campbell, BSc, SFN, SSN, CPT

For more information including quantity discounts, please visit www.ForeverYoung.MD.

DEDICATION

To my main reason for wellness — my family.
You inspired me to get healthy in the beginning and you continue to
support my passion for sharing my story with others.
This journey would not mean nearly as much without your
unconditional love.
May we strive to be forever young together!

ABOUT DR. TORRES

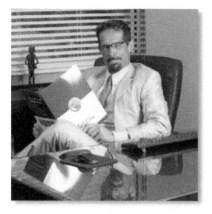

Dr. Torres specializes in the diagnosis and treatment of patients with spine-related pain syndromes and osteoarthritis of multiple joints. He has authored and co-authored several articles published in various medical journals and has also participated in several clinical research studies. His experience is vast:

- University of Puerto Rico (Cum Laude, BS Biology)
- University of Puerto Rico School of Medicine (MD)
- Veterans Administration Hospital, San Juan (Residency)
- Louisiana State University (Musculoskeletal Fellowship)
- American Academy of Physical Medicine and Rehab. (Member)
- American Association of Electro-Diagnostic Medicine (Fellow)
- International Spinal Injection Society (Member)
- American Board of Physical Medicine and Rehabilitation (Cert.)
- American Board of Electro-Diagnostic Medicine (Certified)
- American Board of Pain Management (Certified)
- International Spinal Injection Society (Certificate in Discography)
- Florida Academy of Pain Management (Past Vice President)
- Osteoporosis Program of Florida Spine (Current Director)

Dr. Torres is also the President and Medical Director of ForeverYoung.MD. As a trained age-management physician, he works with patients on preventing age-related disease in order to optimize health and longevity.

ABOUT GABE TORRES

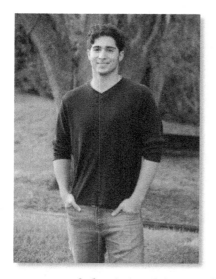

Gabriel – Gabe for short – graduated from the University of South Carolina Beaufort (USCB) where he played four years of baseball. After graduation, he continued his baseball career in Puerto Rico. He is currently a Certified Strength and Conditioning Specialist for professional baseball.

Gabe lends his expertise to ForeverYoung.MD where he helps patients implement lifelong nutrition and exercise habits. He is also in the process of obtaining his certification as a Performance Enhancement Specialist.

TABLE OF CONTENTS

12 - TRY OUR TASTY RECIPES FOR FAT LOSS 111

"Don't let your subconscious habits become your fate. Consciously do the things that will make you healthy, fit, and happy."

~Dr. Torres

CLIENT TESTIMONIAL

When Karen Johns, 73, stepped inside the Florida Spine Institute for a medical appointment, she could not help but notice Dr. Torres' ForeverYoung.MD brochure. No stranger to weight loss programs, Karen was skeptical. She had tried countless programs and points, as well as eating packaged meals. Nevertheless, she struggled to keep off the weight. Karen had fallen victim to "yo-yo dieting." For some reason, that day she decided one more weight-management program couldn't hurt.

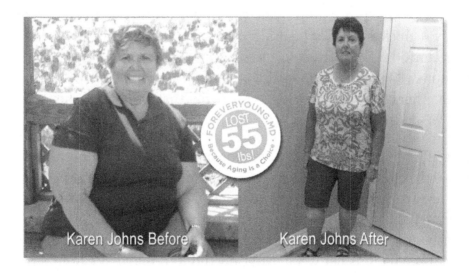

Karen Johns Before   Karen Johns After

What Karen did not expect was the different approach to weight loss ForeverYoung.MD implements with each patient. Karen began a once a week meeting program with Dr. Torres and his team. She quickly discovered that ForeverYoung.MD was dedicated not only to her weekly weight loss goals but to her weekly health.

Dr. Torres started Karen's program with education. Unlike other programs which had spelled out stale meal plans or shipped prepackaged junk with little to no explanation, the staff at ForeverYoung.MD educated Karen on the importance of limited sugar and increased proteins. They didn't just give her the "what." Instead, they explained the "why." That knowledge proved powerful.

Karen was immediately impressed by the ForeverYoung.MD program. For the first time, she discovered how to manage her weight using lasting healthier alternatives in her everyday life. She was finally able to bid good riddance to the short-lived quick fixes she had relied on in the past. With ForeverYoung.MD, Karen describes a newfound confidence in going out to eat with friends. She can enjoy time with her husband and her friends anywhere because she now knows how to eat. Menu choices and thoughtful modifications give Karen the opportunity to stay on track with her goals and stay in the loop with her loved ones.

Not only did the program provide Karen the knowledge she needs to modify recipes and order healthier at restaurants. It adjusted for her medical needs. This knowledge was never addressed with previous programs which left Karen feeling abandoned while piecing together health information to create a diet that would help her shed the pounds.

The staff at ForeverYoung.MD is medically trained and equipped to run tests and examine some of Karen's underlying medical conditions. They are also professionals who also have the ability to modify the program to her individual needs. This combination allowed her to flourish with her customized program and keep a steady weight loss of about three pounds per week. Not only did Karen love the numbers on the scale, but she was pleasantly surprised by the new numbers on her clothing tags as well! Karen has gone down three dress sizes so far and she happily proclaims that the inches off her waist have kept her just as satisfied as the pounds off the scale.

Today, Karen enjoys a once-a-month program focused on keeping the fat off rather than raw numbers. She emails Dr. Torres with questions in between meetings and is constantly thinking of new modifications for her cooking. She tries to pass these lessons and innovations on to her fellow friends who are also ForeverYoung.MD clients. Karen looks forward to continued weight loss and, more importantly, sustained health well into the future.

REFLECTION, STRENGTH, AND INSPIRATION

Several years ago, I made the decision to transform my body and achieve fitness and health excellence. This was a decision that has defined the future course of my life. Today – seven years later – what seemed so distant is a tangible reality. I can, in all honesty, say that I have taken control of my life and have come to realize that the possibilities are endless. The transformation, both physical and emotional, that has occurred in the last seven years is truly amazing.

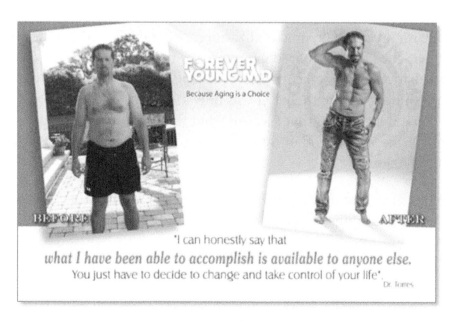

FOREVER YOUNG.MD
Because Aging is a Choice

BEFORE   AFTER

"I can honestly say that
what I have been able to accomplish is available to anyone else.
You just have to decide to change and take control of your life".
Dr. Torres

Struggles Growing Up

Very vividly, I remember the feeling of frustration and inadequacy while growing up. My overweight problem affected my relationship with others and kept me from participating in my favorite sports.

During adolescence, I struggled with low self-esteem and lack of confidence that was the direct result of my physical appearance. I still remember the pain of not been able to take my shirt off in public without embarrassment.

Later on, as an adult and in spite of my low self-image, I overcame some of my fears. I went on to achieve significant milestones in my professional and personal life. However, none of those accomplishments gave me the satisfaction that I gained after successfully completing my transformation.

My Wake Up Call

When I saw life passing me by, along with the disappointments of life, I realized I needed to do something. My desire to change was greatly fueled and made tangible only after seeing myself in an emergency room facing a cardiac catheterization.

Along with my own personal realizations, the tragedy and devastation in my patient's lives bothered me more due to their lack of exercise and poor nutrition. As a medical doctor, it is common for me to evaluate the health of my patients. Yet, it was only after my personal realization in the emergency room that I feared what the future would hold for me. Their lives became constant reminders, and I knew I needed to make a drastic change.

All personal breakthroughs occur when we clearly know the reason why we want to accomplish a specific goal. I truly believe this was the case for me.

My Passion for Fitness

In my 40s, I developed a passion for fitness and nutritional excellence.

During my transformation process, I have completed several half marathons, as well as an Ultra Marathon. I've even won first place in bodybuilding competitions.

All my fitness accomplishments wouldn't have been possible without strenuous strength training. I continue to be active with TRX® Suspension Training which is a form of exercise that develops strength, balance, flexibility, and core stability simultaneously. It is a program developed by the United States Navy Seals.

In addition to my love for fitness training, my lifestyle changed in many other ways. Good nutrition, quality sleep, and stress management also became part of my protocol for a healthy body and life.

Though it wasn't easy in the beginning of my transformation process, every difficult change was worth saving my life as I can now enjoy it with the ones I love.

Where My Strength Came From

I remember the day when one of my four sons approached me with an interesting question. He asked, *"Dad, why do you want to become stronger?"* I had to think for a moment before answering. After all, it was important for me to define the forces behind my motivation to transform my physical condition.

Through the innocence of my young son, I answered him with plenty of good reasons. First, I told him that transforming my physique was an important goal for me as I wanted to be healthy. I went on to explain to him that being in control of my health was not only taking part of my physical wellbeing but also part of taking control of my life. Finally, I explained to him that I wanted to push myself beyond my limits as it empowers me to be better at everything I do in life.

During my transformation, the love and support of my wife and children only strengthened our family bond, and my goals also became theirs. Our common cause has made us closer than ever. But, it was their support that gave me the strength from within to succeed in my goals.

Being an Inspiration to Others

Over the past several years, people have noticed my physical and emotional transformation. I am flattered when they tell me that I have become their role model.

Becoming an inspiration to my family, friends, co-workers, and clients is very heartening. The one thing I can communicate effectively to others is that what I have been able to overcome and accomplish is available to anyone else.

> *"For any change to be of true value,*
> *it has to be lasting and consistent."*
>
> ~Anthony Robbins

The key is to set goals, develop a practical plan, and then uncompromisingly use all resources available to work on this plan. Setting goals that are measurable and attainable is the foundation for getting healthy – as well as for all success in life.

If you are reading this book, you probably have a desire to lose weight and get healthy. Just remember that desire is the first step towards success. Along with desire, persistence and commitment will move you towards reaching your goals. All three are key elements in achieving excellence and success.

Enjoying the Process

Throughout my transformation process, I have learned that accomplishing a goal is not the only thing that matters. In fact, part of what counts is the gratification and excitement endured along the way towards succeeding any goal.

My own transformation has sculpted both my physical body and my character. It has given me the desire to help make this world a bit better by sharing what has helped me to become stronger, healthier, and happier. Enjoying your own transformation process may also enlighten you.

On the Road to Inspiring Others

Finding ways to help others has always been my inspiration in life and the reason why I became a physician. There is nothing that can compare to the exhilarating feeling of making a significant contribution or accomplishing a major objective in life.

Without a focused source of positive change, life quickly loses its flavor. However, pursuing an objective that is worthwhile will test your limits of endurance, solidness of convictions, and strength of character. It did with me! And, it becomes an exciting adventure that can benefit you, your family, and your circle of influence.

Every life properly lived is a beacon that others can follow. I am convinced that I became a winner in life when I wholeheartedly embraced this belief:

"Any goal in life is attainable when you believe it is yours."

I am blessed with four sons that fill my life. If my legacy for them was only a passion for a healthy life that allows them to reach their inborn potential, I consider my efforts worthwhile. I would like to look back at them and see a better world just because I lived a life full of passion, energy, and enthusiasm.

Healthy living that includes fitness and nutrition are an integral part that and has helped a simple dream become a tangible reality. You too can make your dreams a reality.

Warmly,

Francisco M. Torres, MD

Getting Started

Surviving a Slow Metabolism

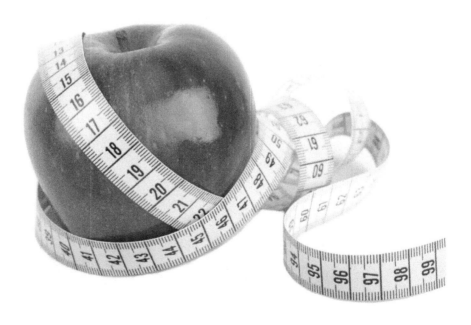

YOU AREN'T TOTALLY RESPONSIBLE FOR GAINING WEIGHT

That's right! While you may have overeaten or eaten foods that cause fat gain, you aren't totally responsible for your eating habits. This may seem strange coming from both a physician and a coach. After all, we have been told time and again that weight gain is the result of unhealthy eating and lack of exercise. Hopefully, you'll see where we're coming from after looking at the bigger picture.

If you lived between the years of 1960 to 1980 as a teen or adult in the United States, you most likely remember the difference in human body size from those who lived then to those who live now. In the last few decades, the overweight and obesity rates have skyrocketed. During the 1960s and 1970s, the overweight population stayed level and was much smaller than today. In fact, only 4.8 percent of men and 7.9 percent of women were considered obese in 1980.[1] That number may even be exaggerated as calculations for being overweight or obese were much more conservative back then than they are today.

Currently, over 75 percent of men and 67 percent of women are considered either overweight or obese.[2] That equates to about 180 million adults in America. Overweight and obese children are also on the rapid rise. Since 1970, obesity rates have more than quadrupled for small children (ages 6 to 11) and tripled for older children (ages 12 to 19).[3] In just 25 years, the United States has become a fat and unhealthy nation.

It may be easy for the medical and health community to urge the overweight and obese community to eat right and exercise. However, the problems behind the rapid growth of an unhealthy nation isn't as simple as blaming lifestyle habits. If you look behind the scene, you'll see a much bigger problem contributing to our unwholesome society.

The Gold Standard for Nutrition Guidelines

In 1992, nutrition education came into effect with the United States Department of Agriculture (USDA) Food Guide Pyramid. Most licensed doctors, dieticians, and other professionals considered this particular nutrition guideline to be the gold standard. It soon became the most widely recognized in the world and was used by those seeking nutrition counseling. Health and nutrition teachers also used this guideline to teach children.

The original hierarchical pyramid presented itself with six food groups with daily recommendations of servings[4]:

1. Grains (breads, cereals, rice, and pastas) – 6 to 11 servings

2. Vegetables – 3 to 5 servings

3. Fruits (including fruit juices) – 2 to 4 servings

4. Proteins (meats, poultry, fish, dry beans, eggs, and nuts) – 2 to 3 servings

5. Fat, oil, and sweets – use sparingly

Unfortunately, the USDA Food Guide Pyramid of 1992 was hugely flawed. Breads, cereals, rice, and pastas were touted as the healthiest foods while fats were vilified as an evil greater than sweet candy. What experts didn't realize was that exaggerated amounts of unhealthy processed grains and a lack of proteins and dietary fats would create a fat society. From the time the nutrition guideline was introduced in 1992 to the beginning of the new decade in 2010, obesity rates nearly doubled in 36 states and more than doubled in 12 other states.[5]

Because the USDA guidelines became a nutrition bible to most professionals in the medical and health fields, patients and clients became loyal consumers of the new guidelines. While they filled their plates with unwholesome fattening foods that ultimately padded their bellies, the scientific community was reporting the injustice of the American diet.

Later, science strongly supported a wholesome diet with more protein and dietary fats while limiting starchy carbohydrates such as grains. In 2005, the USDA revised their guidelines and renamed it *My Pyramid*.

Grains were reduced to half of the original rule. Fruit juices were de-emphasized. Dietary fats now had a place in the pyramid. While a reduction in grains and an increase in fats were improvements to the original 1992 plan, imperfections remained. Proteins were reduced, and serving sizes for certain food groups were not defined.

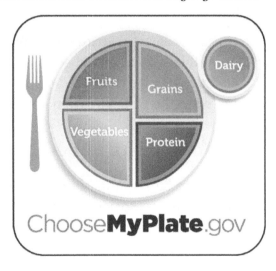

A few years later (2011), the USDA revised their guidelines yet again. The triangular food pyramid was replaced with the *My Plate* model. To your right is a diagram of a dinner plate that was split into four uneven quadrants with vegetables and fruits taking up half the plate.

Grains and protein make up the other half, with a larger emphasis on grains. A cup above the right-hand side of the plate represents the need for milk. Unfortunately, this model also fails in its recommendations:

- It FAILS to provide recommendations for individuals with different goals (i.e., weight gain, weight loss, etc.).

- It FAILS by recommending too much milk. Scientific research has shown multiple risks for a high percentage of the population who have an allergy or intolerance to lactose.

- It FAILS to educate individuals on healthy food types such as whole grains versus processed carbohydrates (i.e., white flour, breads, pastas, etc.).

- It FAILS to provide nutrition information relating to activity levels.

- It FAILS to provide information on supplementation value and its benefits to health.

The USDA made great strides to improving nutritional guidelines, even if it has still fallen somewhat short of the mark. However, the damage was already done to American society as consumers had become acclimated to the USDA's original nutritional recommendations.

Why Most Health Foods Cause Addictions

In addition to flawed nutrition guidelines, food manufacturers have contributed to a fat society. Although their advertisements are ubiquitous, the food industry in reality doesn't have to work very hard to attract customers.

With the hustle and bustle of modern living, people are just too tired to cook. Therefore, pre-packaged foods are a convenience. Dining out also makes it easy for moms who are too tired to cook when they get home from work.

While food manufacturers have made life easier for most Americans, what consumers don't realize is the danger that comes with simple eating. Some know that pre-packaged snacks and fast foods can add to body weight on the scale. However, manufacturers are using certain ingredients in their products – including those labeled "healthy" – that are actually not healthy for you. Some of these ingredients include:

- refined sugar
- high fructose corn syrup
- monosodium glutamate (MSG)
- aspartame

While some are used as flavor enhancers and sweeteners, most are used as preservatives. Nearly all have addictive and harmful substances. You may ask why food manufacturers do this, and the answer is unfortunate. Business is about profit. As long as you are a loyal customer, they get to line their pockets and stay in business.

When Diets Cause Metabolic Decline

If you're like most Americans, you've probably read and tried at least one or two weight loss diets over the years. You may even be reading this book in hopes that you might unlock the secret to losing fat (stay tuned—you'll get something better). Don't feel bad. Most dieters have tried some form of low-carb, low-fat, or other type of diet without much success.

Regrettably, modern technology has fostered the proliferation of bad information – especially when it comes to good nutrition and exercise. It can be quite confusing for someone who just wants honest information.

Unfortunately, most diets are a "one size fits all." They don't take the time to personalize the diet for different body stats (i.e., age, weight, height, activity level, etc.). Instead, all are put on the same calorie diet which is usually dangerously low at 1,000 calories or less. Many diets are also very imbalanced where protein or fats are the emphasis. Other diets may emphasize all vegetables and fruits. However, your body needs a variety of nutrients, and balance is very important.

Summary

The USDA, food manufacturers, and diet literature play a huge role in the American obesity epidemic. Fortunately, you have one book in your hands with excellent information that will provide you with science-based knowledge on nutrition as well as help to get your body into the healthiest shape ever.

IS YOUR METABOLISM IN JEOPARDY?

Have you ever heard someone say, "I have a slow metabolism, and that is why I gain weight so easily"?

A healthy metabolism is one of life's essential ingredients. After all, your metabolism is you. That's right! Your metabolism is how your body does what it needs to do. Trillions of cells make up your body, and these cells are damaged and destroyed each day by wear and tear. Thankfully, your metabolism knows how to repair and regenerate these cells. It is responsible for creating new antibodies, enzymes, neurotransmitters, hormones, other cellular chemicals, and energy to help you perform.

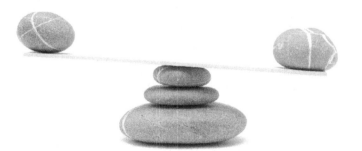

When your metabolism is balanced, you are healthy. However, it is out of balance when you're overweight, sick, and tired. Your metabolism has two sides. One side is the "building up" side and the other is the "tearing down" side. To be healthy, both sides must be in balance. Eating nutrient dense foods builds your body up, and normal daily activities and exercise tear down your body. However, excessive tear down occurs when you don't eat well, exercise and sleep too little, and stress too much.

Often times, constant dieting – as well as yo-yo dieting – damages the basal metabolic rate (BMR). Due to the damage, weight loss becomes difficult. Some can't lose weight at all. Other people may have recently gained weight or have tried to lose weight on their own without success. Unfortunately, strict dieting for a long time can be a detriment to your metabolism. This creates an imbalance that is sometimes difficult to recover from without proper guidance (which you will find in the coming chapters).

If your metabolism is imbalanced for a long period of time, you have an increased risk for something called *Metabolic Syndrome*. With this condition, your risk for health problems rise.

Know the Physical Symptoms

Metabolic Syndrome is a cluster of conditions that increases your risk for serious health conditions such as diabetes, heart disease, and stroke. The cluster may include[6]:

- increased blood pressure
- abnormal cholesterol levels (high triglycerides and low HDL)
- high fasting blood sugar level
- excess body fat around the waist
- damaged BMR[7]

Having just one of these conditions does not mean you have Metabolic Syndrome. However, your risk does increase if you have more than one condition. Even without Metabolic Syndrome, your risk for a serious disease is still increased with just one of these conditions.

Know the Risk Factors

The following factors increase your chances of having Metabolic Syndrome:

- **Age** – Affects 40 percent of the people over age 60.

- **Race** – Hispanics and Asians.

- **Obesity** – Apple shape physiques or those with greater waist lines.

- **Diabetes** – Gestational diabetes during pregnancy or a family history of type 2 diabetes.

- **Other Diseases** – Increases with cardiovascular disease, non-alcoholic fatty liver disease, or polycystic ovary syndrome.

Other Names for Metabolic Syndrome

You have Metabolic Syndrome if your doctor has diagnosed you with any of the following conditions:

- Dysmetabolic Syndrome
- Hypertriglyceridemic Waist
- Insulin Resistance Syndrome
- Obesity Syndrome
- Syndrome X

Summary

Your metabolism is you. Extended imbalances can wreak havoc on your body and promote Metabolic Syndrome. Optimal nutrition will correct faults and help your metabolism towards a healthy state. Our upcoming meal plans will help you.

HOW YOU CAN SURVIVE A SLOW METABOLISM

If you have a slow metabolism – or even Metabolic Syndrome – you probably won't feel your best. You may even have a difficult time losing weight. This is not the time for you to give up. In fact, you need to put all your effort into making some lifestyle changes to repair your body before you move towards full-blown metabolic damage that can affect your nervous, hormone, and immune systems.

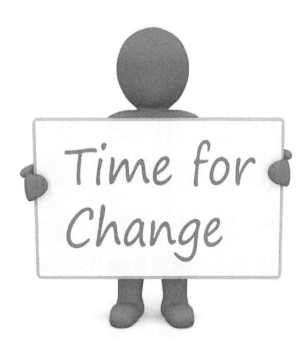

Healing & Jumpstarting Your Metabolism

To get you started on the road to recovery, we're going to teach you what to do so that you can heal and jumpstart your metabolism. Lifestyle changes are necessary for your metabolism to run optimally and your body to function efficiently. With these lifestyle changes, you will lose body fat too!

In Part I of this book, you will learn the five aspects of healthy living that will get you started on the road to recovery and losing body fat quickly:

1. Nutrition
2. Exercise
3. Quality Sleep
4. Stress Management
5. Personal Assessment

For some of you, these changes will be simple. Or, you may have to work a little harder to make these changes if you who have led a life of bad habits. All in all, you can do it. If you don't think you can, then check out the testimonies of those who will change your mind:

- Arthur Boorman – a disabled veteran who is able to walk again and even do backbends.

- Nick Scott – a paralyzed young man who is now a fitness pro, professional ballroom dancer, and author (and still in a wheelchair).

- Ernestine Shepherd – the world's oldest lady bodybuilder who started her healthy lifestyle at the age of 56 and is now 78 years young and aging very gracefully.

Calculating Your "Happy Target Zone"

If you're seeing a practitioner for weight loss, he or she may calculate your calorie needs. If not, you will have to personally calculate them. To do so, knowing your basal metabolic rate (BMR) is important.

Finding Your BMR

BMR measures how many calories you burn at rest. It is the minimum amount of energy expenditure when you are not active, but you are still burning due to heart rate, breathing, and even thinking. It does not include any daily activities like moving around, working, exercising, etc. The calculation is based on your age, gender, and body composition.

You will notice that your BMR result will decrease weekly as you lose weight simply because it takes less effort on the part of your body to function. Obese people actually burn more calories at rest because their bodies are working harder. That is why they lose weight faster when they first diet, while leaner people lose more slowly. As a drawback, obese people can have a heart attack more easily since their heart is working so hard to pump blood to all parts of their body. That is also why it is so much easier for an overweight person to sweat more.

The Harris-Benedict equation includes models for both men and women and will help you determine your BMR:

Calculating BMR for Men

$$\begin{aligned}
& 66 \\
+\ & (6.23 \times \text{weight in pounds}) \\
+\ & (12.7 \times \text{height in inches}) \\
-\ & (6.8 \times \text{age in years}) \\
=\ & \text{BMR}
\end{aligned}$$

Calculating BMR for Women

$$655$$
$$+ \quad (4.35 \text{ x weight in pounds})$$
$$+ \quad (4.7 \text{ x height in inches})$$
$$- \quad (4.7 \text{ x age in years})$$
$$= \quad \text{BMR}$$

Determining Your Total Daily Energy Expenditure

Before determining your daily nutritional needs for weight loss, we first need to determine your calorie needs or total daily energy expenditure (TDEE) for maintaining your current weight. To figure your TDEE, you will multiply your BMR with your activity factor.

Calculating Daily Calories

BMR (Basal Metabolic Rate) _____

Activity Factor Adjustment   x   _____

Maintenance Calorie Needs   =   _____

Activity Factor

1.2	=	Sedentary (little to no exercise; desk job)
1.375	=	Lightly Active (1-3 days per week)
1.55	=	Moderately Active (3-5 days per week)
1.725	=	Very Active (6-7 days per week)
1.9	=	Extremely Active (2x day exercise; physical job)

Finding Your "Happy Target Zone" for Fat Loss

Once you know how many calories you need to maintain your weight, we can easily find your daily nutritional needs or "Happy Target Zone" by subtracting enough calories to ensure you will lose weight. A safe amount is usually between 500 to 1,000 calories per day. The sum will then determine your calorie needs for weight loss which will help you determine which meal plan to follow.

Calculating Daily Fat Loss Calories

Maintenance Calorie Needs   =   _____

Weight Loss Adjustment   -   _____

Daily Calories for Fat Loss   =   _____

Starting the Healing Process with Good Nutrition

In Part II, you'll find our cutting edge meal plans so that you can get started on healing your metabolism right away. Not only will you learn about good nutrition based on science, you'll also learn how to turn nutrition into your own medicine. That's right! Nutrition is actually the best medicine for your body.

Our entire plan includes natural whole foods in balanced proportions that will heal and jumpstart your metabolism. You will include nutrient-filled proteins, carbohydrates, and fatty acids. Proteins will come from many animal sources. However, we will provide options for vegans as well. Carbohydrates will include mostly vegetables, so gear up if you haven't been eating them! You'll enjoy them on our plan as we'll show you simple ways to fix them to be tasty. You'll also get to enjoy fruits on our plan – especially metabolic boosting berries. Grains will be eaten in moderation during certain phases. Dietary fats are extremely important to your metabolism, so we'll also include them – mostly sources with high Omega-3s.

As you look over the lists of food that we've included, you'll find that some are not comprehensive lists. Foods that contribute to sensitivities and allergies in a high percentage of the population (such as dairy and gluten) will be eliminated during our 28-day induction phase. However, some of these foods will be reintroduced in the post-induction phase.

In Part III, you'll find a well-rounded list of tasty and healthy recipes that are simple to incorporate in your diet. You'll also learn when buying organic produce is best, as well as what foods build up your body.

Summary

A healthy lifestyle will help you heal your metabolism, boost your energy, and make you feel your best. You can do that with good nutrition, exercise, quality sleep, stress management, and ongoing personal assessments. Please remember that it does take time to heal your metabolism, especially if you've been excessively tearing it down for a while. Just don't give up hope. By sticking to our plan consistently, you will see positive changes in your body.

Part I

An Integrative Approach to Healing Your Metabolism

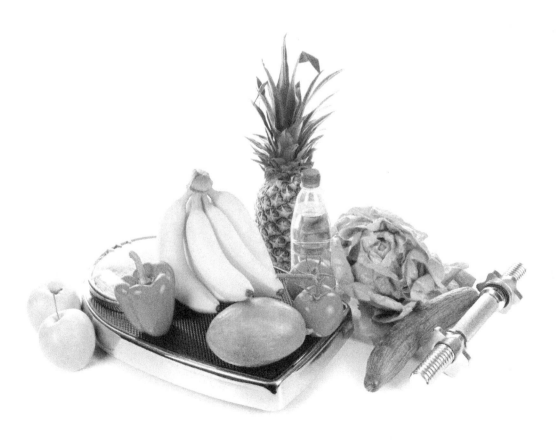

Flush Toxins with Nutritional Medicine

Nutritional Medicine is the practice of preventing and treating disease by providing optimal amounts of substances that are natural to the body. Nutrients such as proteins, carbohydrates, fatty acids, vitamins, minerals, and water are all natural substances your body needs to function properly. Without them, your biological function is disturbed. This imbalance then leads to symptoms and disease. It can even lead to a difficult time losing weight.

The good news is that Nutritional Medicine is able to address your body's imbalances, optimize your health, and help you lose unwanted body fat. It does this through cleansing your system and flushing toxins – all the gunk that has been weighing you down and making you sick.

In Part II, you will find our therapeutic meal plans to be very effective in relieving various symptoms as well as putting you on the weight loss fast track. But before we get into that, we would like for you to understand how each segment of Nutritional Medicine works to heal your body.

Proteins

Protein is a very important nutritional building block for your body. It keeps your blood's pH levels balanced, maintains proper hormone levels, and regulates proper fluid balance. In times of dieting, it preserves muscle and is an energy source when no carbohydrates are available. Your immune system relies on protein for proper functioning.[8] Protein is also very beneficial for weight loss:

> **Higher Metabolic Rate.** Protein is thermogenic and will help you heal your metabolism. It also burns at least twice as many calories as carbohydrates and fats, which provides you with greater fat loss.[9]

> **Increased Glucagon.** Protein increases glucagon which is a hormone that helps you fight the effects of insulin. Unregulated insulin levels will wreak havoc on your body leading to potentially severe health problems. Glucagon also helps decrease the making and storing of body fat, which also means higher fat loss during dieting and less fat gain while overeating.[10]

> **Growth Hormone Regulation.** Eating enough protein ensures your body is getting all the amino acids it needs. Amino acids are the building blocks to making growth hormones. If you don't get enough growth hormones, your metabolism slows down which can lead to lower bone density, muscle loss, and a number of other physiological and mental issues.[11/12]

> **Increased IGF-1.** Protein increases IGF-1 which is an anabolic hormone that increases muscle growth. Higher IGF-1 spares your muscles while dieting.[13] *Ladies – no worries! You only have a fraction of testosterone compared to men, so you won't get big and bulky from eating protein.*

> **Anabolism.** Eating protein keeps your body in an anabolic – building up – state. If you don't get enough protein, your muscles can deteriorate. Since muscle tissue helps you burn body fat, protein is important.[14]

> **B Vitamins.** Many animal protein sources provide a rich volume of B vitamins (especially B12 and B6) which provides you with energy, heals your metabolism, and helps you lose weight.

For optimal health, you should have protein at every meal and snack. Examples of protein include lean meats, chicken, turkey, fish, seafood, egg whites, Greek yogurt, and cottage cheese. When possible, opt for organic or wild-caught.

Vegetables & Fruits

If you're not fond of vegetables and fruits, you're going to start loving them! They provide your body with a plethora of nutrients and antioxidants that you just can't get from other food types. By consuming a diet high in vegetables, you are lowering your risk for chronic conditions such as type 2 diabetes, heart disease, and cancer.[15/16] Additionally, they will help you lose weight for a variety of reasons:

> **Fewer calories provide weight loss.** Because vegetables and fruits are lower in calories, you can eat more and stay satiated longer than if you were eating foods higher in calories.[17]

> **Increased water and fiber provide fullness.** Vegetables and fruits have a high water and fiber content. The impact of water adds weight to these foods without increasing calories. Plus, fiber helps you lose weight.[18]

> **Fiber eliminates waste.** Fiber in vegetables and fruits provide healthy bowel function as it keeps food moving through your digestive tract. This encourages quicker elimination which boosts your overall gut health and reduces fat and cholesterol in your bloodstream.[19]

> **Fiber is indigestible.** Your body cannot digest or absorb fiber. Therefore, the calories you get from the fiber in vegetables and fruits are not processed.[20]

> **Blood sugar is stabilized.** Vegetables, and fruits in the right serving sizes, have a low glycemic index which help sustain blood sugar levels and insulin concentrations. This enhances satiety, energy, and body composition.[21]

➢ **Vitamin C heals metabolism.** While vegetables and fruits have a plethora of vitamins, many have a rich source of Vitamin C which helps to heal your metabolism.[22]

Vegetables and fruits are packed with nutrients – vitamins, minerals, and phytonutrients – that will help protect your body from destruction. Green vegetables are extremely important for cleansing your system so try spinach, kale, and watercress. Berries are also an excellent fruit as they are high in antioxidants and low in sugar; they will protect your body from pollutants.

Whole Grains & Legumes

You've probably heard that whole grains like wheat and oats are healthy. However, not all whole grains are created equal. In fact, some whole grains actually digest as quickly as sugar-filled candy bars, if not quicker. Recent studies have proven that even wheat is not as complex as it was once thought to be.[23] During weight loss, you want to stay away from any carbs that raise blood sugar extensively and increase the risk of inflammatory responses. This includes tubers (potatoes), oats, and gluten-filled grains like wheat, barley, and rye.

Because starchy carbs – even in their natural state – are loaded with calories, it's best to keep them at a minimum for health and weight management. Though research shows that whole grains protect against heart disease, other studies have shown that whole grains contribute to insulin sensitivity and Type 2 Diabetes.[24/25] This is especially true when eaten in excess. For those who are sedentary and overweight, starchy carbs (especially the refined types) are likely to cause metabolic damage and store fat when overeaten.[26]

Therefore, nutrient timing of natural starchy carbs is of utmost importance for metabolism and weight management. Starchy carbs are best utilized when you are active and should therefore be limited to after strenuous exercise as they help your body to recover faster by replacing energy stores.[27/28] Think of them as a reward for following your exercise plan.

Because it's easy to overeat starchy carbs, it's best to limit them for when they are needed. You will be receiving the best carbohydrates in your diet through vegetables and fruits which will provide your body with a plethora of vitamins, minerals, and other nutrients. The best grains include those that are gluten-free such as amaranth, quinoa, and brown rice. Legumes may include a variety of beans, lentils, and peas.

Healthy Fats

Contrary to what you've been told about dietary fat in the past, it is not your enemy. In fact, your body requires and depends on natural fatty acids. So, forget about the fad diets of the past, and eat more natural foods containing them.

Natural dietary fats are an important source of energy as they help[29]:

> ➢ balance your hormones,
> ➢ promote a healthy immune system, and
> ➢ keep inflammation low.

In fact, they are important to every single cell in your body. If your cell membranes are full of unhealthy *gunky* fat, nutrients cannot pass through to truly detoxify your body. A variety of natural fats will keep your body and brain running optimally. The healthiest fats to include in your diet are Omega-3 fatty acids, olive oil, and coconut oil.

Omega-3 Fatty Acids

Omega-3 is a powerful nutrient that will detoxify and heal your metabolism by knocking out the bad fat and toxins from your body. It will heal your metabolism so that you can lose body fat.

This very special fatty acid converts into compounds much more potent than the actual fatty acids – 10,000 times more potent.[30] These compounds help bring inflammatory responses in the body to an end. Research has shown that Omega-3 fatty acids can heal and prevent many diseases such as heart disease, high cholesterol, high blood pressure, diabetes, cancer, rheumatoid arthritis, osteoporosis, macular degeneration, Alzheimer's, and mental illness.[31/32/33/34] It has even been proven to reduce body fat by improving insulin sensitivity and using stored body fat for energy when combined with a healthy diet of lean proteins, vegetables, and fruits.[35/36]

The easiest way to include Omega-3 in your diet is to eat cold-water fish that is wild caught such as salmon, tuna, mackerel, herring, and sardines. Nuts and seeds such as walnuts, flaxseeds, and chia seeds are also high in Omega-3s. You may also supplement with a quality fish oil product.

Olive Oil

The health benefits of olive oil are unrivaled as research reveals more benefits of this special fatty food nearly every day. Even the world's longest-living cultures include a relatively high level of dietary fat which are mostly from extra virgin olive oil.

The beneficial effects of olive oil have been widely studied and could be due to the phytochemicals it contains which also include anti-inflammatory properties. A recent study published in *The Journal of Nutritional Biochemistry* confirmed the importance of including olive oil in the diet when exercising.[37]

Instead of eating processed salad dressings, make a point to include extra virgin olive oil in its place. Just mix it with red wine vinegar, garlic, and your favorite spices for a delicious healthy dressing. You can also add it to your cooked vegetables as a flavor enhancer.

Coconut Oil

You may have heard of coconut oil's miraculous benefits in recent years. Research has shown it to be an extremely valuable antidote for many health conditions due to its antioxidant and anti-inflammatory action. It is also metabolized in the body differently than other fats such as olive oil. In fact, the body doesn't store coconut oil as it does other fats. It uses energy immediately and is very helpful for weight loss.[38]

Include coconut oil in your diet, especially when cooking as it holds up to high heat much better than olive oil. You may also find it in supplementation form.

Water & Herbal Teas

If you've been drinking caffeinated and sugar-filled beverages, it's time to stop if you want to heal your body. Sodas and fruit juices contain quite a bit of calories from refined sugar that raise your blood sugar levels. But, replacing them for zero-calorie sodas can be a huge mistake.

While you may think you're doing yourself a favor by reaching for the lesser of two evils, sugar-free sodas are processed with chemically laden and addictive substances like aspartame. These chemicals alter your metabolism in such a way that can make you sick and fat.

Research has even shown that the sugar and additives used to sweeten soda are much more addictive than cocaine.[39] Whether it's sugar or sugar-free, they both are dangerous to your metabolism and weight. Water and decaffeinated herbal teas are your best source for healing your body and losing weight.

Water

We want you to consume water as your main beverage choice as it helps facilitate every metabolic process in your body. Water is so essential to your body that you need at least half your body weight in ounces – and sometimes more if you are very active. Why so much water? Your body is actually made up of nearly 60 percent of your total body weight. That's a lot of water, so you want to make sure you're replenishing what makes up your body. Water benefits you in variously important ways[40]:

> ➤ carries nutrient and oxygen to your cells
> ➤ protects organs
> ➤ moistens mucous membranes
> ➤ lubricates joints

> ➤ regulates body temperature
> ➤ helps the kidneys and liver by flushing out waste products
> ➤ helps prevent constipation

Recent studies have also shown that water is your secret weapon to losing weight. Just by drinking two cups of water prior to each meal helps you lose more body fat than if you didn't drink those two cups.[41]

Herbal Teas

Research has shown that some tea and coffee beverages are beneficial to your body. This is due to the polyphenols or natural chemicals classified as having antioxidant, anti-viral, and anti-inflammatory properties. Polyphenols protect your body from free radicals that cause damage.

Green tea is especially beneficial as it has been shown to prevent and inhibit cancer growth; protect against heart disease, diabetes, and DNA damage; and boost immunity.[42/43] Numerous studies have also shown that green tea plays a role in decreasing body fat by increasing energy expenditure and fat oxidation.[44]

Other than green tea, there are many exciting herbal teas on the market that are beneficial for a variety of reasons. You can choose from dandelion, chamomile, mint, and more. Ginseng and green tea are especially good for weight loss. If you opt for an herbal tea, be sure it's decaffeinated as caffeine is off limits in our 28-day induction phase. Also try organic as many tea plants are sprayed with pesticides which wreak havoc on your metabolism.

Summary

Nutritional Medicine is very beneficial for treating fat loss. Saturating your cells with vitamins, minerals, and phytonutrients will also cleanse and optimize your body for better health.

ADDING THE RIGHT EXERCISE AMOUNT FOR GOOD HEALTH

Use it or lose it! You may have heard that expression before, and it's very true when it comes to your body. If you don't use it, you will surely lose it as your body depends on you moving it to stay healthy. Your muscles become weak, your joints become stiff, and your heart won't function efficiently without physical activity. Inactivity can be as dangerous as cigarette smoking!

Research shows that after the age of 30, the average decline in resting metabolic rate with each passing decade is three to 8 percent.[45] Muscle loss occurs with this metabolic loss. On average, five pounds of lean muscle mass is lost per decade after the age of 30. However, exercise can deter this loss with other healthy lifestyle choices such as diet, stress management, and quality sleep.

Benefits of Exercise

Because muscle is so metabolically active, its loss is directly responsible for much of the metabolic loss. Therefore, it should be clear that age isn't responsible for metabolic decline. Rather, inactivity is a huge factor. It's important to protect muscle mass as you grow older as you'll also preserve your resting metabolic rate. Other than protecting your muscles, exercise provides you with several other benefits[46]:

> ➤ burns more calories

> ➢ detoxifies the body
> ➢ reduces stress
> ➢ promotes better sleep

While these four health benefits are crucial for weight loss, a combination of cardiovascular and resistance exercise also provides many other health benefits[47]:

> ➢ better glycemic control
> ➢ lower triglycerides
> ➢ improved circulating lipids
> ➢ improved blood pressure
> ➢ decreased inflammation
> ➢ reduced carotid intima-media thickness progression

Additionally, exercise may even save your life. Recently, the World Health Organization identified physical inactivity as the fourth leading risk factor for global mortality. It follows right behind hypertension, tobacco use, and hyperglycemia.[48]

Exercises You May Enjoy

If it's a structured program, make sure it is one that you can easily incorporate into your daily routine, and ease into that routine as you don't want to burn out before you've really given yourself a chance to get started. Following are some great exercise regimens you may want to try. Find one that you enjoy and exercise regularly. If you've never exercised, or are sedentary, start with at least five to 10 minutes per day for five days per week. Once you've started this healthy habit, it will become easier throughout the coming weeks.

> ➢ structured exercise programs (weight or resistance training)
> ➢ water aerobics or swimming
> ➢ recreational or leisure exercise
> ➢ yoga

Two Important Types of Exercise

Science proves that not all exercise is created equal. In fact, there are some approaches that yield better results than others. For instance, you need to know which exercise is best for burning fat if your goal is to lose weight. While the answer may not be simple, knowing how each type of exercise – aerobic versus anaerobic – works with your body will help.

Aerobic Exercise (Cardio Training)

Aerobic exercise – also termed *cardio* – increases your body's functional capacity to transport and use oxygen. Aerobic exercise requires oxygen from the blood to fuel energy-producing mechanisms of your muscle fibers. This type of exercise is usually light activity that can sustain you for a long period of time. Examples include running and cycling.

For cardiovascular benefits, both the American Heart Association® and the British Heart Foundation recommend at least 30 minutes of moderate-intensity aerobic activity at least five days per week. For additional health benefits, they also recommend moderate to high intensity aerobic activity at least two days per week.[49]

Anaerobic Exercise (Resistance Training)

Anaerobic exercise – also termed *resistance training* – greatly increases your body's functional capacity for developing explosive strength. Anaerobic exercise usually includes short-term activity that is typically high intensity. Oxygen consumption is not sufficient to supply energy demands being placed on your muscles. This type of exercise requires bursts of activity for short periods of time like sprinting and weightlifting.

Resistance training is important for reversing loss of muscle function and structure, as well as joint weakness, associated with age and chronic illness.[50]

Aerobic or Anaerobic for Fat Loss?

Both aerobic and anaerobic exercise boost metabolism and burn body fat. The key is to include both types of exercise into your workout. Aerobic exercise increases your endurance and cardio health while anaerobic exercise helps you to gain and maintain lean muscle mass. Lean muscle mass is needed to burn fat.

Including exercises that incorporate both aerobic and anaerobic segments are the perfect balance to your workout regimen and provide you with the benefit of maximum fat burn. You can include both types separately by alternating days for each, or you can incorporate training that utilizes both segments together such as swimming, kickboxing, or circuit weightlifting.

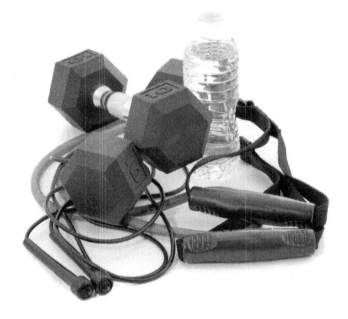

Cardio Exercise & Examples

To help you get started with aerobic exercise, we're providing two examples below. Both are structured for moderate to high intensity cardio conditioning. So, go ahead and give it your best effort. Start with Example #1 and work yourself up to Example #2 over the course of several months. Perform these exercises every other day with 30 minutes of moderate-intensity walking, swimming, or other exercise in-between those days.

Cardio Example #1

3 MINUTE WARMUP (INTENSITY LEVELS 2-4/10)
 	
START CIRCUIT
 	
    → 1 minute (intensity level 5/10)
    → 1 minute (intensity level 6/10)
    → 1 minute (intensity level 7/10)
    → 1 minute (intensity level 8/10)
    → 1 minute (intensity level 9/10)
 	
REPEAT CIRCUIT TWICE
 	
1 MINUTE (HIGH INTENSITY LEVEL 10/10)
 	
2 MINUTES COOL DOWN (INTENSITY LEVEL 2-3/10)
 	
TOTAL 11-21 MINUTES

NOTE: Beginners may want to start with one circuit and work up to three circuits over the course of a few months.

Cardio Example #2

3 MINUTE WARMUP (INTENSITY LEVELS 2-4/10)

START CIRCUIT

> → 1 minute (high intensity level 8-9/10)
> → 1 minute (low intensity level 3-4/10)

REPEAT CIRCUIT UP TO 6 TIMES

5 MINUTES (LOW INTENSITY LEVEL 3-4/10)

20 MINUTES (MEDIUM INTENSITY LEVEL 5-6/10)

3 MINUTES COOL DOWN (INTENSITY LEVEL 2-3/10)

TOTAL 33-45 MINUTES

NOTE: Choose circuit repetitions based on your exercise level: beginners do 2-3 rounds; intermediates do 4-5 rounds; and advanced do 6-7 rounds.

Resistance Training & Examples

Many people think of bodybuilders when they hear the term *resistance* or *strength training*. However, resistance training is important for every human body. Though it may include lifting dumbbells and barbells, there are many different types of resistance training:

> ➤ weight machines using weights with hydraulics
> ➤ medicine or weighted balls
> ➤ kettlebells
> ➤ resistance bands

> ➢ body weight

Because resistance training may be new to you, we're including a few important pieces of information before you get started. When lifting or resisting weights, be sure to use safety precautions. Also, it's best to warm your muscles prior to training, as well as stretch afterwards.

Safety with Resistance Training

Whether you are a beginner, or one who has been a pro for years, it's important to pay attention to safety when performing resistance training. By paying attention to good form, you'll reduce your risk for injury. If you're not sure where to begin, ask your gym's wellness coordinator or physical exercise trainer to help you get started.

Warmups

Before beginning any resistance training exercises, you will need to warm your muscles so they are able to handle the upcoming stress from exercise. Start with a light cardio session such as walking, cycling, or rowing. Warmups should last five to 10 minutes.

Performing Exercises

A typical resistance training program for a beginner may include 8 to 10 exercises that work the major muscle groups of the body. Each exercise should comprise of 8 to 12 repetitions. Training sessions should be completed two to three times per week.

Stretching

After completing resistance training, you should always perform stretching exercises for about 10 to 15 minutes. Because resistance exercises can cause your muscles to shorten, stretching counteracts that shortening while promoting flexibility and allowing your muscles and joints to move through their full range of motion. This keeps your body limber by releasing muscle tension and tightness.

Allow Muscles to Recover

Your muscles need time to repair and grow after a workout. Allowing sufficient rest in between resistance training workouts is important. A 48 hour period is sufficient for recovery time.

And, for you ladies – NO WORRIES! Your muscles cannot physically get big and bulky like those of men. You only have a fraction of the hormone *testosterone* which allows muscles to get really big. Therefore, your muscles will get toned and tighter allowing for a more slender body.

Preventing Plateaus

If you do the same activity all the time, your body is likely to plateau and you won't see changes as quickly. After several weeks, your body adapts to the exercises you're doing and won't offer you the same benefits as they once did. Therefore, changing your routine every four to 8 weeks will keep your muscles challenged. Changing your exercises will also keep your muscles guessing and your results coming.

Training Major Muscle Groups

Train all major muscle groups of your body. After all, you don't want to just do all upper body exercises. Have you ever seen a guy who has large chest and arm muscles with scrawny legs? Obviously, he neglected to work on his lower body. We don't want you toppling over due to imbalance. Therefore, we encourage you to strengthen and improve your entire body and keep all your muscles in balance for best performance. By focusing on a balanced body, you'll gain the following benefits:

> ➤ prevent injuries
> ➤ improve posture
> ➤ avoid aches and pains
> ➤ promote a proportionate body

Resistance Training Plan Example

To lose body fat the quickest, do full body circuit training. You may find a workout plan on the next page to get you started. By completing this combination exercise, you'll kill two birds with one stone – both cardio and resistance training. By performing circuits three times per week, you only have two days of cardio left.

Start with Circuit #1 until all sets are completed. Do one set for each exercise with the appropriate amount of repetitions, and do not rest between exercises until you've reached the end of the last exercise in the circuit. Then rest two minutes, and repeat the circuit two more times. Once all sets for the circuit have been completed, move to Circuit #2 and then Circuit #3.

You may want to schedule your training sessions for Monday-Wednesday-Friday or Tuesday-Thursday-Saturday. This allows your muscles to rest and repair before the next workout session.

Beginners may want to start with one set and work up to three sets over the course of several months. If you aren't familiar with any of these exercises, please refer to YouTube as they provide a vast array of videos for every exercise under the sun. You may also ask a wellness coach at your gym to help you.

See the circuit training example on the next page.

Circuit Training Example

CIRCUIT #1 – UPPER BODY EXERCISES

→ Dumbbell Bench Presses – 3 sets x 8-12 reps
→ Wide-Grip Lat Pulldowns – 3 sets x 8-12 reps
→ Standing Shoulder Presses – 3 sets x 8-12 reps
→ Seated Dumbbell Curls – 3 sets x 8-12 reps
→ Bench Dips – 3 sets x 8-12 reps

CIRCUIT #2 – LOWER BODY EXERCISES

→ Machine Squats – 3 sets x 8-12 reps
→ Romanian Deadlifts – 3 sets x 8-12 reps
→ Dumbbell Glute Kickbacks – 3 sets x 8-12 reps
→ Standing Calf Raises – 3 sets x 8-12 reps

CIRCUIT #3 – ABDOMINAL EXERCISES

→ Stability Ball Crunches – 3 sets x 15-25 reps

Stretching Exercises

As mentioned previously, stretching for at least 10 to 15 minutes after cardio or resistance training is important to your body. Following are a few good stretches. Hold each stretch for 15 to 30 seconds each. Repeat as desired. You may also find these stretching exercises on YouTube if you don't know how to do them already. Most gyms will also have wall charts that show you how to stretch.

➢ overhead stretch
➢ chest and front shoulder stretch
➢ triceps stretch
➢ cat stretch

> ➢ on your side quadriceps stretch
> ➢ seated hamstring and calf stretch

Summary

For best overall health benefits, a combination of cardio and resistance exercises is necessary. If you aren't currently exercising, we encourage you to include regular physical activity. According to the American Heart Association®, health benefits increase with at least 30 minutes of moderate-intensity exercise five days per week.[51]

You may also find better success in your workouts by keeping a journal. Just get a notebook and write down the exercises you plan to do. Take it with you to the gym, and mark off the items as you do them. Make notes where you feel you need to improve, and circle items where you've had a personal best. Also check out exercise apps for your phone to better plan and take notes. Let your journal motivate you to be consistent.

MANAGING REST & STRESS LEVELS FOR BALANCE

Some periods of our lives are smooth sailing. Without the stress, our body's organs – and the chemicals they produce– are in balance. However, living in a state of *Utopia* is not an everyday reality for most of us. Whether it's personal, financial, work-related, or a combination of some or all, stress can spin us out of control like cars on a slick highway.

Under normal stress, your hormones can put you back on track and get you headed down the right path again. Within moments, they can help you navigate through life again whether it is lifting a bad mood, breaking a fever, or reducing pain.

While our bodies are intelligent and know just how to produce enough hormones to protect us from physical or emotional stress, excessive stress can wreak havoc on your chemical messengers. In turn, this causes other chemical messengers to fail to do their jobs efficiently. Heart rate, blood pressure, body temperature, sleep, pain perception, immune system response, and metabolism can all be negatively affected. Inflammation and weight gain may even occur. Applying techniques to reduce or manage stress and help you sleep may reduce cortisol levels that cause weight gain.

Stress Management Techniques

Although stress can take its toll on you, you can decrease its damaging effects by practicing methods to reduce it. Finding the right strategy is key. You may find taking a walk in the country works well for you, but your best friend may find a hot bubble bath in candlelight works better. Just knowing you have the power to control your own stress with the right strategies is a stress reducer in itself. Our clients have found some of the following Mindfulness-Based Stress Reduction (MBSR) techniques to calm their stress triggers. You may also find they work for you as well.

Focus and Breathe

Two techniques you may use to manage stress are *Diaphragmatic Breathing (DB)* and *Progressive Skeletal Muscle Relaxation (PSMR)*. In DB, consciously inhale deeply through your nose and exhale through your mouth at the same time you are expanding your diaphragm. With PSMR, visualize a word, phrase, or image that you feel is relaxing. With your entire body – from head to toes – tighten, hold for a few seconds, and then release groups of muscles one at a time. You may want to start from the top of your body and move down towards your toes, or vice versa. With this technique, do several sets until you are relaxed.

Release Negativity

Another MBSR technique can release your negative of self-defeating thoughts and help you into relaxation. For those who can't sleep, this technique works especially well. Also, become aware of any self-defeating thoughts. Stress ignites with negative thoughts as we gain weight, acquire pain, and grow older. Try this technique if you're saying things like "I'm too fat" or "I just can't lose this weight." To try this technique, get into a comfortable position and close your eyes. As the negative or self-defeating thought comes to you, imagine it drifting off like a cloud or sailing down a stream until you can no longer see it.

Keep a Journal

You can reduce stress and release any negative emotions like anger and anxiety by keeping a daily journal. A study conducted by the Southern Methodist University found that people feel a purpose and make positive life changes when they spend 20 minutes writing in a journal about their emotional circumstances. [52]

Exercise

When stress starts to build, a short brisk walk or meditative exercise such as yoga can relieve stress. One study published by the *Annals of Behavioral Medicine* suggests 90 minutes of yoga reduces perceived stress and cortisol levels.[53] With a little determination, you too can find benefits through yoga. Try meditative or relaxing types of yoga like Hatha, Vinyasa, Iyengar, or Restorative.

Better Sleep Techniques

Stress and worry can cause pain as your cortisol levels rise. Following are some techniques that may help you relieve your stress for better sleep. Additionally, you may want to check your lifestyle choices as well. Are you drinking caffeinated beverages or napping during the day? Might your medication schedule be causing restless nights? By eliminating these factors as well as including the given techniques, you may be able to finally get the rest you've been longing for.

Relax Your Face

Tighten all your facial muscles and hold for two seconds. Take a deep breath. Relax muscles while exhaling. Repeat a few times.

Buy a Memory Foam Pillow

You can purchase memory foam pillows for your neck, your back, and your hips. Once you've found the most comfortable position, you don't have to fight with your pillow each night.

Space Your Fitness Routine

Spread your exercises out instead of cramming your weight training, cardio, and other exercises into one session. Never overextend yourself as the rising cortisol levels from strenuous exercise will only increase your stress. Cortisol is your stress hormone.

Meditate

Visualize your worries and imagine them being carried off downstream until they disappear over the horizon. Continue doing this with all your worries until you are just relaxing near a soft flowing stream. Listen to the flow of water and the birds singing. Smell the nearby flowers, and feel the warm sun shining down on you. Relax.

Take a Hot Soothing Bath

A soothing hot bath before bedtime may relax you. Use candlelight instead of overhead lightbulbs. Add soothing essential oils, along with Epsom salts. The aromatherapy from the essential oils will help relieve your stress levels, while the salts will pull toxins from your body. Together, they will put you into a relaxing state for sleep.

Summary

Applying stress management techniques, as well as getting quality sleep, will help protect your body. Along with other healthy lifestyle choices, your metabolism will begin to heal. Then you'll find it's much easier to lose weight and be healthy.

SEEKING HELP & PROFESSIONAL ASSESSMENTS

Are you someone who is tired of endless diets and still not losing weight? Or, are you someone who depends on prescription medication for weight loss? If you are someone who has had a difficult time losing weight, then you may have an underlying medical condition that is preventing you from losing.

Sometimes, a person's disturbances are so off kilter that a thorough assessment by a physician is necessary. Genetics, environmental influences, and the physical-psychological connection are areas that the physician should explore. However, research proves that 90 percent of chronic illnesses are due to lifestyle choices.

With Nutritional Medicine, a patient is able to attack problems without the limitation of conventional drugs. Along with making lifestyle changes to help the healing process, practitioners may prescribe other protocols that will bring balance to a patient's life whether it is through modern medicine, detoxification and therapeutic diet, nutraceuticals, or stress management.

While many practicing doctors will focus on and treat symptoms, specialized physicians in Nutritional Medicine focus on the *patient*. By finding the root cause(s) of individual biochemistry, practitioners of Nutritional Medicine are able to remove most hindrances that contribute to weight gain. Therefore, you must seek out a qualified

Nutritional Medicine physician if you have been doing all the right things but haven't been successful at losing weight.

Patient Assessment

After a thorough assessment, a qualified Nutritional Medicine practitioner is able to understand how key processes are specifically affecting a patient. These processes occur at the cellular level. They dictate function, repair, and maintenance of the body and even keep the patient alive. They are also related to larger biological functions influenced by genetics and environmental factors.

When these biological functions are disturbed, the body becomes imbalanced which leads to symptoms and disease if not effectively treated. This confused state can affect your:

- immunity
- inflammatory response
- energy levels
- hormone regulation
- structural integrity
- psychological equilibrium
- digestive tract
- assimilation of nutrients
- toxic waste removal

If your body is in a confused state, the good news is that Nutritional Medicine is able to address most clinical imbalances. A qualified physician (and his professional staff) will partner with you so that you can take charge and improve your own health. Together, you and the physician can work on a customized treatment plan with available interventions that provide you with the most impact on your underlying functional needs.

Summary

Rather than treating just the symptoms that may contribute to weight gain, an approach that determines the triggers of those symptoms can actually heal your body. By looking deeper into symptomatic causes, problems can actually be addressed rather than masked. Nutritional Medicine may include nutritional supplements, detoxification and therapeutic diets, and counseling on lifestyle changes. Seek out a qualified practitioner who specializes in Nutritional Medicine.

Part II

Simple Everyday Meal Plans that Help You Lose Fat

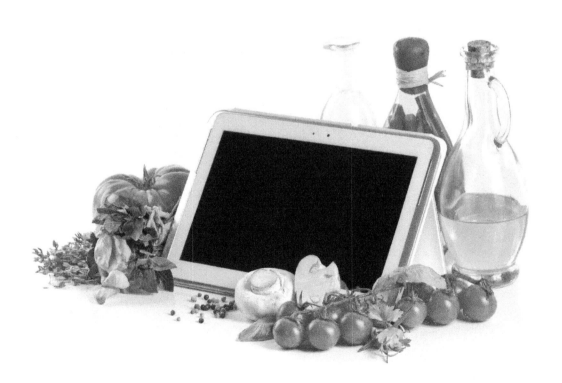

JUMPSTART YOUR METABOLISM IN JUST 28-DAYS

Transformation is about becoming the healthy, productive, and happy person you're meant to be. To help you make your transition to a healthier lifestyle, you will begin your amazing journey by utilizing our innovative and straightforward weight loss plan. Hundreds of our own clients have had incredible success following the steps you'll read in the following pages.

The first step to weight loss is to jumpstart your metabolism. You will do this with the induction phase of our diet plan. All it takes is four weeks to begin losing weight – particularly body fat. Additionally, you will feel healthier in all aspects of your body – physically, mentally, emotionally, and even spiritually.

Our induction phase is a simple approach that will heal and boost your metabolism which is necessary for weight loss. Plus, it will help you regain your energy and feel great. It is a 28-day meal plan geared toward certain individuals:

- people who have dieted all of their lives
- people who suddenly need to lose weight
- people who can't seem to lose weight on their own

Often times, weight loss dieting damages the basal metabolic rate (BMR). Due to the damage, weight loss may become difficult later on.

Some can't lose weight at all while others may have tried to lose weight without success. No matter what your situation, our 28-Day Induction Phase will get you started.

To be successful with our 28-Day Induction Phase, you will need to make a commitment to stick with it. After all, it's only for 28 days and the health benefits you'll receive are worth it. Four weeks is all it takes to jumpstart your transformation and improve your health.

During this phase, you'll exchange some of your old unhealthy habits for healthy ones. These changes will lead to better energy and focus. Best of all, you'll be well on your way to losing unwanted body fat.

After four weeks, you'll be ready to transition to our ongoing weight loss plan. This is our Post-Induction Phase where you'll have more choices in managing your weight. You can read more about it in the next chapter. For now, let's discuss some things you'll encounter with our 28-day Induction Phase.

Breaking the High Carb Cycle

You may have heard that carbohydrates – or "carbs" for short – are bad for you. That statement is true to a certain extent. The fact is that your body responds negatively when certain carbs are eaten. This may include foods made with refined white flour and sugar. It may also include natural starchy carbs such as potatoes and rice, as well as fruits, when eaten in excess.

Because your body can't store large amounts of carbs in the body, it will use carbs as its first source of energy. Upon immediate use, your body will then store small amounts in the muscles and liver to use between meals as a steady source of energy. Any excess amounts will then be stored as body fat.

Not only will you gain body fat if excess carbs are eaten. Eaten on a regular basis, your body will no longer work correctly. In fact, serious health conditions are related to eating excess carbs. Insulin resistance is one of the serious health conditions that may lead to diabetes, heart disease, and cancer. Losing body fat becomes very difficult with insulin resistance.

Therefore, our 28-Day Induction Phase was created to help you break the high carb cycle. You will need to avoid any pre-packaged, processed, and refined foods during the next four weeks. (You may refer to a list of foods to avoid later in this chapter.)

Choosing Healthier Options with Low-Glycemic Carbs

With this phase, you will eat a very clean and low-glycemic diet which will include high quality complex carbohydrates such as dark green leafy vegetables such as kale, spinach, and arugula. Other vegetables may include a rainbow of choices. You may also include one serving of berries per day. By eating these low-calorie nutrient-dense carbs, you will be pumping your body full of vitamins, minerals, and phytonutrients.

By replacing the empty calorie foods with healthy options, you will jumpstart your metabolism. Your cells will be cleansed, and your body will no longer need the extra fat. Your cravings will even diminish.

What to Expect

In the beginning of our 28-Day Induction Phase, you may encounter certain symptoms due to the change in diet. Some do experience intense food cravings in the beginning which are usually due to an addiction to carbs and sugar. Stay the course! These feelings will subside as you fill your body with the appropriate nutrients.

You may also encounter headaches, low energy, and constipation or diarrhea. Your symptoms are normal with diet changes. The severity of your symptoms may depend on how badly addicted you are to carbs. We encourage you to drink plenty of water during this time to flush out the toxins. The sooner the toxins leave your body, the better you will feel.

Foods to Avoid During the 28-Day Induction Phase

Following are foods that you will need to avoid during the 28-Day Induction Phase. While some of these foods will not be re-introduced in the Post-Induction Phase, we will introduce others when we transition to that phase.

High Sodium & MSG Foods:

- canned foods
- condiments (mayonnaise, ketchup, soy sauce, etc.)
- cured meats (beef jerky, sausage, deli meats, etc.)
- snack foods (potato chips, salted nuts, etc.)
- sauces and gravies

Sugary Foods:

- sugar-based drinks (fruit juices, sodas, sweet tea, alcohol, etc.)
- pastries and doughnuts
- cereals
- snack foods (candy, cookies, cakes, ice cream, etc.)

White Flour-Based Foods

- breads, bagels, crackers, croutons
- pastas and noodles
- pancakes and waffles
- cookies, cakes, chips, and other processed snacks

Other Carbs

- corn
- grains and rice
- potatoes

Dairy Foods

- milk
- yogurt
- cheese (including cottage cheese)
- creams (including ice cream)

Hydrogenated & Saturated Fatty Foods

- cured meats
- sausages
- salami & pepperoni
- bacon
- fried meats and eggs
- store-bought salad dressings
- cooking oils (all except coconut and olive oils)

Beverages

- juice (fruit)
- sodas (all – including sugar-free)
- caffeinated drinks (coffee)
- alcohol (beer, wine, and hard liquor)

Keeping Balance with Nutrient-Dense Foods

The key to success for our 28-Day Induction Phase is "balance." You will do this with the right foods. Not only will you eat the appropriate carbs. You will include them with the right proteins, dietary fats, and water. By consuming a balanced diet of all macronutrients, you will be well on your way to optimal health.

To help you stay balanced during our 28-Day Induction Phase, you should include nutrient-filled foods as indicated in the remainder of this chapter.

Protein Foods

As you read in Step 1, proteins are fundamental components of all living cells and are comprised of many substances: enzymes, antibodies, and hormones. For your body to function properly, your body will need healthy protein foods for tissue growth and repair. You will be able to find a variety of proteins from animal and plant sources, and you should include some protein at every meal and snack.

For weight loss, include protein as 35 percent of your total daily calories. An easy way to measure the right amount of protein for you specifically is to use the size and thickness of your palm as a serving. You are getting the right protein amount if you are hungry three to four hours after eating. If you get hungry in two hours or less, you need to include more protein at your next meal. If you are not hungry for five to seven hours after your meal, then you need to decrease the amount of protein at your next meal.

Following are some protein sources you may want to include in our 28-Day Induction Phase. If you can, be sure to choose grass-fed, wild, range-free, or organic.

- lean beef (95% lean or better)
- wild game (venison, bison, veal, etc.)
- pork tenderloin
- chicken or turkey breast
- egg whites
- fish (salmon, tuna, mackerel, herring, sardines, etc.)
- seafood (shrimp, crabs, lobster, etc.)
- organic tofu or tempeh
- hemp hearts/seeds

- protein powder (low-carb and no-sugar added)

Carbohydrate Foods

As mentioned earlier, low glycemic carbs are best to heal and boost your metabolism. Better yet, super foods that are very dense in nutrients will help your body heal faster. A healthier body leads to a faster metabolism which will help you lose weight and feel great.

You may include either cooked or raw vegetables or fruits. Frozen items are fine as some are even better than fresh due to flash-packing. If possible, choose organic. Always pair your carbs with protein and dietary fat. Following are carbs that you may include:

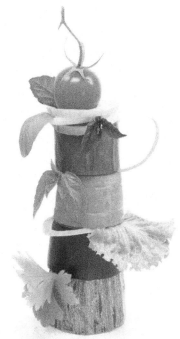

- dark green leafy vegetables (kale, spinach, Swiss chard, etc.)
- cruciferous vegetables (broccoli, Brussels sprouts, cabbage, cauliflower, etc.)
- rainbow vegetables (bell peppers, tomatoes, cucumbers, etc.)
- root vegetables (beets, onions, radishes, sweet potatoes, etc.)
- mushrooms (portabella, shiitake, cordyceps, Lion's Mane, etc.)
- berries (blueberries, raspberries, blackberries, cranberries, and strawberries)
- lemons and limes

Healthy Dietary Fat Foods

While fat got a bad reputation for several decades, research now shows that certain types of dietary fat are actually healthy and essential for the body. Without them, the body is susceptible to inflammation, and the brain is unable to function optimally. In fact, dietary fat ensures the integrity of every cell in the body as it transports important nutrients. The best types of dietary fat include those found in nature:

- oils (fish, olive, flax, and coconut)
- avocado
- nuts (walnuts, pecans, almonds, etc.)
- seeds (flaxseeds and chia seeds)

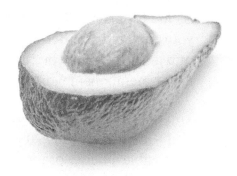

You may also obtain healthy Omega-3 fatty acids in cold-water fish such as salmon, tuna, mackerel, herring, and sardines.

Water & Beverages

The sooner your body flushes toxins, the faster you will lose weight and feel healthier. Water will do this for you. Be sure to drink at least half your body weight in ounces, but we encourage you to try to drink one gallon of water per day. You may also consume the following during our 28-Day Induction Phase:

- sparkling water
- green tea
- herbal teas
- decaffeinated coffee
- low-sodium vegetable juice (as part of a whole meal)
- low-carb protein shake (only 1-2 per day with no sugar-added)

Drop the Fat Food Guide Pyramid

To help you visualize your macronutrient breakdown, please see our nutritional diagram on the next page. Our Drop the Fat food pyramid is a graphic representation developed by our ForeverYoung.MD nutritionist and is an excellent tool to help you make healthy food choices. The food guide pyramid can help you choose from a variety of foods so you get the nutrients you need.

Drop the Fat Food Guide Pyramid

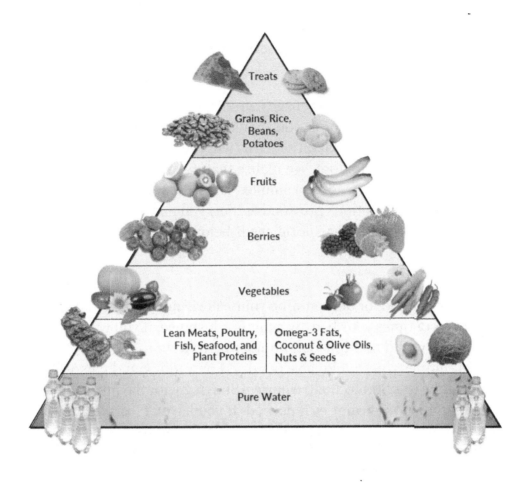

How Many Calories are Necessary on the 28-Day Induction Phase

Let's be honest. Most diets fail because calorie counting is difficult. Who has the time or energy for it? That is why many people either quit or opt for professional help. If you've been unsuccessful, we hope you'll opt for the latter. Professional help may cost a little bit of money, but it can be worth the price if it's a good program.

In our office, we require at least 1,000 calories per day during our 28-Day Induction Phase. Anything less will place your body in a dangerous "starvation" mode where your body will hold onto any stored fat as it thinks that it's in a crisis. By opting for professional help, weekly assessments provide close monitoring. That being said, calorie intake should be based on your body stats – age, gender, weight, height, and activity level.

In our Getting Started section (pages 24-28), we provided an equation to calculate how many calories you should be getting so that you don't enter the danger zone of starvation. This will provide you with your happy target zone for fat loss. We realize that not everyone is great at math, so we are also providing a simpler calculator. If you are having trouble using the equations provided earlier, you may use two easier methods to determine your calorie needs below.

Easier Calorie Calculator

The easiest method for determining your calorie need is to avoid going below 10 to 12 times your body weight. For instance, if you weigh 160 pounds, you would multiply that number by 10 to 12 to find out the range of calories you should have per day. For a 160 pound person, that would equate to 1,600 to 1,920 calories. Starting with the multiplier of 12 allows room to cut calories if needed. If you haven't lost weight within two weeks, then you'll know it's time to cut more calories.

Once you've determined your total daily calorie count, you can then divide that total with the number of meals and snacks you will be eating per day. If that includes five meals, then your calorie count per meal would be 320 to 384 calories if using the example in the last paragraph.

Eyeball Method

If the "Easier Calorie Calculator" method is still too difficult or strict for you, you can actually use the eyeball method. Your body provides you with a pretty nifty tool in counting calories without being so precise.

This tool is your hand. You may use the size and thickness of your palm to determine the cut of protein (beef, chicken, turkey, or fish).

Then fill half your plate with dark green leafy and rainbow colored vegetables for your carbs. Use your thumb for measuring dietary fats such as flax, olive, or coconut oil to add to your veggies. Also, include one serving of berries per day that measure half the size of your fist.

Measuring Tools

Your kitchen scale can actually be your best friend. Measuring cups will help with carb servings while measuring spoons will help with dietary fat servings. And if you're using the eyeball method and not losing weight after a few weeks, then you'll need to seriously consider using one of the equations we've provided to calculate your calories and start measuring your foods if you want to lose weight.

Trial and Error

In the beginning, this plan can involve a little bit of trial and error. That is okay. Nobody is perfect, and learning anything new takes time. You must remember that you just have to keep practicing. If you're not seeing a professional practitioner to assist you, then you'll have to self-assess on a weekly basis. You'll determine whether more changes are needed by monitoring your weight, girth measurements, and how you're feeling.

5 Tips to Help with Your Transition

1) Create a relaxing atmosphere for your eating experience. Turn off the television, computer, and phone. And, don't eat while driving. Sit and enjoy. This practice will help you to connect with your food and help you to feel what is happening to your body while you eat.

2) Take time to chew your food. Savor every bite and reconnect with the joy of eating.

3) Avoid stress while eating. Focus on your food – how it smells, feels in your mouth as you chew, and tastes.

4) Stop eating before you're feeling full. Eat only until you are 80 percent full which is just enough to satisfy your hunger. This allows time for digestion and satiety. Then put down your fork.

5) Eat at planned meal times and do not deviate. Three full meals and two or three snacks per day should allow you to be eating at approximately every three hours. Therefore, you should not need to snack in between. Eating only at your planned meal times is staying mindful.

Your Tracker for Our 28-Day Induction Phase

Week 1   3/15

- Determine your total daily calorie range by using the Harris-Benedict formula on pages 24-28 or the easier calorie calculator on page 70. If you really aren't great with equations, use the eyeball method instead on page 70-71.

- Determine your calorie range for each meal by dividing your total calories by the number of meals you plan to eat each day. Plan to eat every three to four hours minus the time you're asleep.

- Take your multi-vitamin and supplements.

- Drink one gallon of water per day to flush toxins.

- Do not deviate from the diet. ↓ 3 lbs.

3/15 165.8
3/21 163.2
3/29 161.6
4/1 161.2

Week 2

- Do a self-assessment to monitoring your weight, girth measurements, and health.

- Re-determine your total daily and meal calorie ranges if you've lost weight. Continue to eat every three to four hours during waking hours. If you've had any cravings or hunger during the first week, increase your protein intake.

- Continue to take your multi-vitamin and supplements.

- Drink one gallon of water per day to flush toxins.

- Start to get some daily activity. Walking is a great choice as it is easy and you can do it anywhere. You can even walk in place in your own home if you need to. If you can, walk for 15 to 20 minutes per day. Or, you may continue with the exercise you did prior to doing our plan. Just don't overdo it.

- Do not deviate from the diet.

Week 3

- Do a self-assessment to monitoring your weight, girth measurements, and health.

- Re-determine your total daily and meal calorie ranges if you've lost weight. Continue to eat every three to four hours during waking hours. If you've had any cravings or hunger during the first week, increase your protein intake.

- Continue to take your multi-vitamin and supplements.

- Drink one gallon of water per day to flush toxins.

- Increase your daily activity. If you started walking last week, increase your time to 30 minutes per day. You may also incorporate some other form of light exercise.

- Do not deviate from the diet. You are well on your way to a healthier body. Stick to the plan and you will lose weight.

Week 4

- Do a self-assessment to monitor your weight, girth measurements, and health.

- Re-determine your total daily and meal calorie ranges if you've lost weight. Continue to eat every three to four hours during waking hours. If you've had any cravings or hunger during the first week, increase your protein intake.

- Continue to take your multi-vitamin and supplements.

- Drink one gallon of water per day to flush toxins.

- Increase your daily activity. Consider increasing your time to 40 minutes per day. You may also incorporate more strenuous exercise 2-3 days per week. This may include exercises such as weight lifting, basketball, hiking, etc.

- Do not deviate from the diet. If you've been following the program since the first week, you will lose at least five to 10 pounds by the end of this week.

Summary

Congratulations! You should be well on your way to healing and boosting your metabolism and losing some weight by now. You will now move to our Post-Induction Phase where you will continue to lose weight and feel better physically, mentally, emotionally, and spiritually.

6

Continue Fat Loss with Cutting Edge Breakthroughs

If you've just completed our 28-Day Induction Phase, you will find the next step of our program simple. This phase includes our ongoing weight loss plan which is the next step towards your amazing transformation. You will continue a healthy lifestyle through proper nutrition, supplements, exercise, adequate rest, and stress management. It's important that you continue your weekly assessments whether you are doing them yourself or with a professional practitioner.

All the components of our Post-Induction Phase are geared towards helping you build a healthier body so that you can live your life to the fullest. And, when you can live your life to the fullest, you are happier. Living a balanced life in body, mind, and spirit is living a healthy life – one that wards off illness and disease. It is also a life that is energetic and productive. When you're able to do the things you want to do in life, you also set an example for others to live a healthier lifestyle. What can be better than that?

Like our 28-Day Induction Phase, you will need to make a commitment to stick with it. Our Post-Induction Phase is a lifelong commitment, though you will have more food choices than you did during the previous phase.

Adding Higher Glycemic Foods

As you continue to lose weight with our Post-Induction Phase, you will begin incorporating some higher glycemic foods such as dairy, grains, potatoes, fruits, and more. We're sure you'll be excited about this! However, you will follow the same concepts from the previous phase when you eat them.

Incorporating a Treat Day

Even more exciting is that you will be able to have a "treat" day once per week. Your treat day may consist of pizza, spaghetti, or lasagna. It may include a cookie or ice cream for a snack. By including a treat day, the body is constantly guessing so that your weight loss doesn't plateau. Besides, it's nice to enjoy your favorite foods.

Most of our clients include this day during the weekend as this is the usual gathering time with family and friends. It just makes it more enjoyable. Just remember this is not a license to binge and eat to your heart's content. You must still be mindful and control your portions.

If you find that you're not losing weight, you may want to cut back to one sensible meal on your treat day instead.

Continuing Healthy Habit Building

Because you started with our 28-Day Induction Phase, you already know a little about nutrition. You should have a good idea about the kinds of food that boost your metabolism. You may also refer to the previous chapter as needed. We encourage you to continue working on forming good habits to benefit you and your body. Building good habits takes time, but they will become second nature the more you work on them. Best of all, you will continue healing your metabolism.

A Structured Meal Plan that Includes Nutrient Timing

With our Post-Induction Phase, you will find a more structured meal plan. This is a guide that will help you learn what foods are good choices for particular meals. By using nutrient timing, you will have the most benefit for boosting your metabolism, losing body fat, and regaining your health.

On the following pages, you will find groups of foods to use in our menu plan template for our Post-Induction Phase. Continue with this phase for 12 weeks, and adjust if you must. Your weekly assessments will tell if changes are necessary.

Post-Induction Phase Food Groups

Group A – Proteins

Include 30 to 35 percent of proteins in your total daily calories. To figure this amount, use the following equation.

(Body Weight x 10) x 35% = Protein Calories per Day

Example: (160 pounds x 10) x 35% = 560 Calories per Day

You may then determine how many protein calories you will need for each meal by using the following equation:

Protein Calories ÷ Daily Meals = Protein Calories per Meal

Example: 560 Calories ÷ 6 meals = 92 Protein Calories per Meal

Because proteins average 7 calories per gram, you may determine your serving size with the following equation:

> Protein Calories per Meal ÷ 7 grams = Protein Serving Size
>
> Example: 92 Calories ÷ 7 grams = 23 grams per Serving

If you have a food scale, you can measure this out to the exact amount. However, some scales only allow you to weigh ounces. If this is the case, use the following equation:

> Protein Serving Size ÷ 7 grams = Protein Serving in Ounces
>
> Example: 23 Calories ÷ 7 grams = About 3 Ounces per Serving

Below are the proteins allowed on our Post-Induction Phase:

- lean ground beef (5% or less fat)
- London broil
- round steak
- chicken breast
- turkey breast
- egg whites (1 egg white = 4 protein grams)
- fish (salmon, tuna, mackerel, herring, sardines, white fish, etc.)
- organic tofu (1 ounce = 2 protein grams)
- organic tempeh (1 ounce = 5 protein grams)
- hemp hearts/seeds (3 Tablespoons = 11 protein grams)
- ForeverYoung.MD Slim Shake (1 Tablespoon = 8 protein grams)

Group B – Complex Carbohydrates

You may begin adding in some grains, rice, and potatoes that you could not have with our 28-Day Induction Phase. Because many of these foods are high in calories and carbs, be sure to use your measuring cups when dishing these onto your plate. If you find that you have cravings after eating any of these foods, eliminate it and try a different type the next time. A serving size is one-third of a cup.

- brown or wild rice
- plain Old Fashioned oatmeal
- quinoa
- amaranth
- sweet potato or potato (2 ounces)
- teff

Group C – Simple Carbohydrates

In our 28-Day Induction Phase, you were allowed to have a variety of berries. You'll be glad to know that you may begin including other forms of fruit during our Post-Induction Phase.

- apple and pear – ½ small
- apricot – 2
- berries (blueberries, raspberries, and blackberries) – 1/3 cup
- grapefruit – ½
- melon (cantaloupe & honeydew) – ½ cup
- kiwi – 1
- nectarine – ½ small
- orange – ½ small
- plum or prune – 1
- strawberries – ¾ cup
- watermelon – ½ cup

Group D – Fibrous Carbohydrates

Remember that vegetables are your best source for all carbohydrates. If you would like to replace Group B or C with Group D, you are more than welcome to. A serving size is approximately 1 cup raw or ½ cup cooked vegetables. You may have up to two servings per meal. Following includes a list of foods you may enjoy.

- asparagus
- bell peppers
- beets
- broccoli
- Brussels sprouts
- cabbage
- cauliflower
- collard greens
- cucumbers
- green beans
- kale
- lettuce
- mushrooms
- okra
- onions
- radishes
- spinach
- squash
- Swiss chard
- tomatoes
- zucchini

Group E – Dietary Fats

Don't forget your dietary fats. Balancing your diet with healthy sources is extremely important for the health of your cells and function of your body. You will get small amounts of dietary fat from animal proteins, including Omega-3 fatty acids from cold-water fish such as salmon, tuna, mackerel, herring, and sardines. However, you will still need to include extra sources. The best dietary fat sources are Omega-3s, so be sure to include plenty of these. But, please limit nuts and cheese to one or two servings per day.

- oils (fish, olive, flax, and coconut) – 1 to 3 teaspoons
- avocado – ¼ to ½ of fruit
- nut butters (almond, peanut, cashew, etc.) – 1 to 3 teaspoons
- nuts (walnuts, pecans, almonds, etc.) – 1 to 3 Tablespoons
- seeds (flaxseeds and chia seeds) – 1 to 3 Tablespoons
- cheese – 1 slice or 1 ounce

Post-Induction Phase Meal Plan Templates

Post-Induction Phase Weeks 1-4 Meal Plan Template

MEAL 1 – A, B, and E

MEAL 2 – A, C, and 1 TSP. COCONUT OIL

MEAL 3 – A, D, and E

MEAL 4 – A, 1/3 CUP BERRIES, and 1 TSP. COCONUT OIL

MEAL 5 – A, D, and E

MEAL 6 – A and 1 TSP. COCONUT OIL

Post-Induction Phase Weeks 5-8 Meal Plan Template

MEAL 1 – A, B, and E (ADD C FOR FIBROUS CARBS)

MEAL 2 – A, C, and 1 TSP. COCONUT OIL

MEAL 3 – A, D, and E (ADD B FOR COMPLEX CARBS)

MEAL 4 – A, 1/3 CUP BERRIES, and 1 TSP. COCONUT OIL

MEAL 5 – A, D, and E

MEAL 6 – A and 1 TSP. COCONUT OIL

Post-Induction Phase Weeks 9-12 Meal Plan Template

MEAL 1 – A, B, C, and E

MEAL 2 – A, C, and 1 TSP. COCONUT OIL

MEAL 3 – A, B, D, and E

MEAL 4 – A, 1/3 CUP BERRIES, AND 1 TSP. COCONUT OIL

MEAL 5 – A, D, and E (ADD B FOR COMPLEX CARBS)

MEAL 6 – A and 1 TSP. COCONUT OIL (ADD 1/3 CUP BERRIES)

NOTE: Shaded food items are the changes from the previous menu.

Summary

As the end of 12 weeks, you will be well on your way to looking and feeling your best. Many of our clients have experienced a weight loss of up to 30 pounds during this timeframe. Some have even seen more. If you're sticking to the plan without deviation, you too could reach your goals for success. If you still have a great amount of weight to lose, you may continue this 12 week plan.

If you do continue our Post-Induction Phase for more than 12 weeks, be sure to start from the beginning. This will keep your weight from plateauing as you mix up the macronutrient amounts.

When you are ready, you will move onto our Maintenance Phase. Enjoy your start to the finish line!

SIMPLY MAINTAINING YOUR SEXY NEW BODY

If you've reached the Maintenance Phase, we'd like to say "Congratulations!" Over the last four months or so, you've gone through tremendous changes by building healthy habits, losing weight, and getting healthier. This is a great accomplishment, and you should be proud.

However, success does not end there. Statistics do show that more than 64 percent of dieters will regain their pre-dieting weight within two years after weight loss. Reasons may vary amongst those who have regained weight, but the biggest reason is due to emotional issues and food cravings that were not dealt with during the weight loss period. In addition, many don't have a good support system at home. Weight loss can only truly be considered successful if you've maintained your goal weight for two years or longer. To see real benefits then, it's important to stick to your healthy habits. After all, this is a very critical time in your weight loss journey.

Readjusting Your Meal Plan

During the Post-Induction Phase, you learned what foods are healthy options to help you lose weight. However, these same healthy foods are the ones that will keep you at your maintenance weight and living healthy for a lifetime. The only difference is that your serving sizes will need to be readjusted so that you don't lose too much weight. Therefore, we have a new meal plan template for you to follow over the course of the next four to 8 weeks.

Every other week, you will increase your calorie intake by 100-150 calories until you've reached your sweet spot for maintenance. This will allow your body time to adjust to the new calorie intake without weight gain rebound. Please note that you do not have to follow the meal plan template all the way out to 8 weeks. If you find that you are regaining weight at week 6, then you need to go back to week 4 and stay there for maintenance. Please find your new meal plans on the following pages that will help you move towards maintaining your weight. You'll find shaded food items that indicate changes from your previous menu plan for weight loss.

Maintenance Plan for Weeks 1-2

By doubling the complex carbs in meal 1 and coconut oil for meal 6. This will provide you with an additional intake of 100 to 150 calories. This two week adjustment is just enough so that your weight won't rebound.

Maintenance Plan Weeks 1-2
Meal Plan Template

MEAL 1 – A, B X 2, C, AND E (DOUBLE THE COMPLEX CARBS)

MEAL 2 – A, C, AND 1 TSP. COCONUT OIL

MEAL 3 – A, B, D, AND E

MEAL 4 – A, 1/3 CUP BERRIES, AND 1 TSP. COCONUT OIL

MEAL 5 – A, B, D, AND E

MEAL 6 – A, 1/3 CUP BERRIES, AND 2 TSP. COCONUT OIL (DOUBLE THE COCONUT OIL)

Maintenance Plan for Weeks 3-4

For weeks 3 and 4, you will double your fruit serving size for meal 2 and complex carbs for meal 5. This is an additional 100 to 150 calorie step-up from the previous two weeks.

Maintenance Plan Weeks 3-4 Meal Plan Template

MEAL 1 – A, B X 2, C, AND E

MEAL 2 – A, C X 2, AND 1 TSP. COCONUT OIL (DOUBLE THE FRUIT)

MEAL 3 – A, B, D, AND E

MEAL 4 – A, 1/3 CUP BERRIES, AND 1 TSP. COCONUT OIL

MEAL 5 – A, B X 2, D, AND E (DOUBLE THE COMPLEX CARBS)

MEAL 6 – A, 1/3 CUP BERRIES, AND 2 TSP. COCONUT OIL

Maintenance Plan for Weeks 5-6

If you still need to add calories to maintain weight, you can do that with meals 3 and 5 by doubling complex carbs and dietary fat. Again, these additions will increase your calories by 100 to 150.

If you find you are teetering between the last meal plan and this one, then you can cut your added calories by half for both complex carbs and dietary fats.

Maintenance Plan Weeks 5-6
Meal Plan Template

MEAL 1 – A, B X 2, C, AND E

MEAL 2 – A, C X 2, AND 1 TSP. COCONUT OIL

MEAL 3 – A, B X 2, D, AND E (DOUBLE THE COMPLEX CARBS)

MEAL 4 – A, 1/3 CUP BERRIES, AND 1 TSP. COCONUT OIL

MEAL 5 – A, B X 2, D, AND E X 2 (DOUBLE THE FAT)

MEAL 6 – A, 1/3 CUP BERRIES, AND 2 TSP. COCONUT OIL

Maintenance Plan for Weeks 7-8

For weeks 7 and 8, you may exchange the berries in meal 3 for another fruit if you'd like. However, you may keep the berries. Just double the serving size for whichever fruit you choose. For meal 5, you may double the dietary fat.

Again, watch your calories. If you are teetering the scale, then you may want to decrease your added fruit for meal 4 or complex carbs for meal 5 by half.

However, if you still need to increase your calories after week 8 for maintaining your weight, use your best judgment as to where you need to add calories.

Please find your maintenance plan for weeks 7 and 8 on the following page.

Maintenance Plan Weeks 7-8
Meal Plan Template

MEAL 1 – A, B X 2, C, AND E

MEAL 2 – A, C X 2, AND 1 TSP. COCONUT OIL

MEAL 3 – A, B, D, AND E

MEAL 4 – A, C X 2, AND 1 TSP. COCONUT OIL (EXCHANGE BERRIES FOR DOUBLE FRUIT)

MEAL 5 – A, B X 2, D, AND E (DOUBLE THE COMPLEX CARBS)

MEAL 6 – A, 1/3 CUP BERRIES, AND 2 TSP. COCONUT OIL

Ongoing Evaluation

By now, we hope you've experienced the type of transformation you can be proud of. After all, you are well on your way to a healthy lifestyle. If you find that you are ever regaining weight, evaluate your habits. It's simple to go back to our meal plan templates to get you back on track. Just stay mindful and you will reach success.

Reintroducing Old Foods

Additionally, you may begin adding a few foods that were not allowed on our plan. Just use common sense when it comes to ingesting these foods. For instance, caffeine can be useful and alcohol may be pleasurable. However, common sense will tell you that having more than two or three servings is inappropriate for your weight loss success and health.

Also, you may want to try adding one food back in over the course of two or three days to see how your body responds to it. This will tell you if you may have an intolerance or allergy to it. If you reintroduce too many foods at once, detection will be harder. Just remember to use your intelligence – not your emotions – in making the best decisions when it comes to food.

Summary

Our 8 weeks of meal plan templates for maintaining weight will help you reach the calories you need in a natural and easy way without disrupting your biological rhythms. Once maintenance is reached, you will need to stay the course as it takes a full two years to be truly successful at weight loss. If you do find that you have a weight rebound, you may always come back to our plans to help you get back to where you need to be.

In the next chapter, we have included a section for athletes. Because athletes have a strict nutrition schedule for times they are competing, they sometimes have eating and weight problems during their off-seasons. If you're someone who has opted for training and competing, please read Step 8 to help you stay optimally healthy.

In Part III of this book, you will find some interesting information that may help you along your transformation journey. We have even included some tips that will help you towards success, as well as some delightful and surprising foods that enhance your health. We also provide you with a list of foods that pose a danger to your health unless you opt for organic. You will even find an extensive chapter of delicious recipes that will help you during and after your journey.

WINNING THE GOLD – NUTRITION TIPS FOR THE ATHLETE

This chapter may not apply to every dieter, but we want to include a few tips for those in the competitive field of athletics. Nutrition is extremely important for the athlete if he plans on being at the top of his or her game. High performance requires quality nutrients – vitamins, minerals, and phytonutrients – for energy expenditure and recovery. Therefore, we are including some helpful tips to keep shining athletes winning the gold.

Demanding Sports Demand Good Nutrition

Most sports require a demanding schedule for athletes. For instance, the baseball player performs in 140 games within 152 days. Their game consists of quick short bursts of close to maximal output or strength with long rests in between. With the exception of pitchers, most baseball players are not running for extended periods of time and do not need to load up on carbohydrates like marathon runners. However, baseball players still need to consume sufficient amounts of carbs due to the length of the games and the amount of time spent performing throughout the day as well as the year.

A Typical Day in an Athlete's Life – Sample

Diet within sports is based on the simple goal of enhancing and/or maximizing performance – not just for games but also for practice.

While many people think athletes only perform in games, a typical day of performance is actually 8 hours or longer. As an example, take the minor league baseball player whose typical day ranges from 8 to 13 hours:

Typical Day of a Minor League Baseball Player With a 7 PM Game

10:30 – 11:30 AM – STRENGTH TRAINING

1:00 PM – REPORT TO FIELD FOR EARLY WORK

3:00 – 4:45 PM – BATTING PRACTICE BEFORE GAME

7:00 – 10:15 PM – GAME

As you can see, the total time spent working is 12.5 hours in one day. Multiply those hours by the 142 games in one season. The total equates to the same amount of hours of a typical 9 to 5 job in half the weeks. That's right! The athlete works the same amount of hours in 22 weeks that a typical corporate worker does for 44 weeks. Besides the time worked, the athlete is under extreme pressure which increases their stress levels. This is why nutrition is critical for the athlete. Nutrition can make the difference in a team starting hot or ending cold.

It's About Performance, NOT Aesthetics

While most people who focus on diet and nutrition are those who want to have a well-built physique or for health purposes, the athlete is focused on it purely for performance. Following are key nutrition factors for the athlete. Because these factors are generalized, each athlete should personalize them to fit their needs accordingly.

Protein

Most protein consumed should be lean animal protein such as steak, chicken, and eggs. However, this is not always possible due to the limited amount of resources at times. Therefore, quality protein shakes and bars are alternative options.

The recommended protein intake for the athlete should be higher than the normal recommended daily intake (RDI). While the normal adult RDI is 0.8 grams per pound of bodyweight, athletes should consume about 1.5 to 2 grams of protein per pound of bodyweight due to the daily high energy demand on their bodies. Most athletes perform for extended periods of time and demand extra nutrition to support that as well as recovery.

Carbohydrates

Carbohydrates are a key component to an athlete's performance but are often overlooked because of their bad reputation for weight gain. However, they are an essential energy source that supplies the athlete high levels of energy. Most carbohydrates should come from vegetables, fruits, and starchy carbs.

The athlete should consume anywhere from 2.25 to 4.5 grams of carbohydrate per pound of bodyweight. Endurance athletes such as long distance runners will require more and therefore be on the upper end of intake. Those on the lower end of intake include sprinters, skilled, or strength athletes.

Fats

Dietary fats provide the athlete's body with several benefits: energy, insulation and protection, as well as the formation of healthy cell membranes. Most importantly, they are critical for providing energy during exercise or activity – especially for lower intensity types.

Keeping this in mind, the athlete needs to strive for a balance when it comes to dietary fats. Combined with starchy carbohydrates, too much fat can lead to cardiovascular disease and/or diabetes. Dietary fat intake should equate to about 20 to 35 percent of total daily calories.

Water

Drinking enough water cannot be stressed enough for athletes of all ages. Drinking when thirsty is not sufficient. The athlete must consume water well before, during, and long after performance. It is critical for performance as well as injury prevention.

Two hours prior to activity, the athlete should consume about 16 ounces of water. During activity, 6 to 8 ounces should be consumed every 15 to 20 minutes. After activity, 20 ounces for every pound of bodyweight lost will replenish the athlete and keep him well hydrated.

For long lasting sports, sports drinks are an option. However, the athlete needs to be careful to choose his beverage wisely as many sports drinks contain high amounts of sugar which cause blood sugar levels to spike and fall.

Summary

Nutrition is critical for the athlete. Therefore, planning a food budget is also important for the athlete. While some organizations and teams do have their own budget set aside for athletes, this is not true for all. Many young athletes have little resources for the necessary nutrition their bodies need and therefore suffer physically. Their game suffers as well. What athletes put into their bodies is an underappreciated and crucial part of any team's success.

Part III

Important Tips & Recipes to Help You Lose Fat

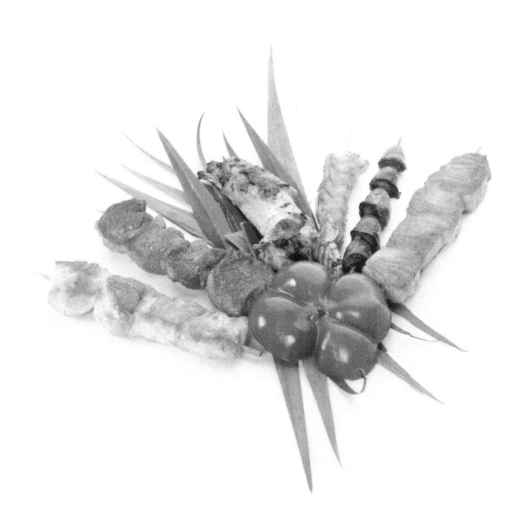

USING 21 TIPS FOR SUCCESSFUL WEIGHT LOSS

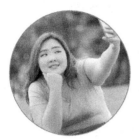

Take photos of yourself before starting the plan. Let these selfies be a motivation to continue with your transformation efforts. Every four weeks, take new photos. By comparing your progress, you will see changes that will continue to encourage you to reach your goals.

Eat balanced meals and snacks each day. Include protein, carbohydrates, and dietary fat throughout the day to stabilize blood sugar and hormonal shifts that usually result in food and sugar cravings. See meal plans.

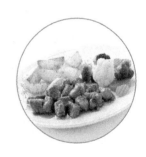

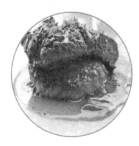

Include enough protein in your daily meals. Your protein intake should be about 35 percent of your daily calories. Be sure you get protein in with every meal and snack. Your body requires healthy protein foods for tissue growth and repair.

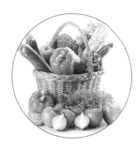

Combine nutrient dense carbohydrates with proteins. Low glycemic super foods are very nutrient dense and will help your body heal faster which leads to a faster metabolism. Vegetables are the best source of carbohydrates, so be sure to fill your plate with plenty.

Add healthy dietary fat to your meals. Certain fatty acids will help reduce inflammation and heal your body. They will also help you lose unwanted body fat and reach your transformation goals quicker. Include Omega-3 fatty acids, olive oil, and coconut oil.

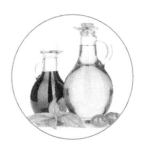

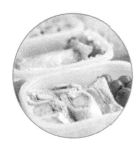

Plan and prepare your meals ahead of time. With work and extra-curricular activities, you can easily pack prepared meals. Don't have time to prepare? Be sure to select healthy options at your favorite restaurants or buy something already prepared at the deli of your local supermarket.

Make your snacks simple with protein shakes. To make planning meals easier, include protein shakes mixed with water or unsweetened almond or coconut milk. Drink them twice per day for your snacks. They are quick, easy, and extremely convenient when you're on the run.

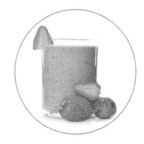

"Our daily decisions and habits have a huge impact upon both our levels of happiness and success." ~Shawn Achor

Eat a snack before dining out. Waiting for food at a restaurant or family function can make you overly hungry. This can cause you to overeat when food is presented. So, eat a small snack before heading out so you don't overeat.

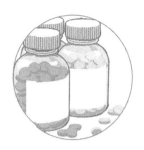

Ask your waiter for a customized meal. Tell your waiter that you are highly allergic to different foods. Ask for lean, grilled meat or fish without added oil. Also, ask for steamed vegetables without any added oils or butter. Add your own olive oil in the right portion.

Drink water every day. Your minimum goal should be one-half your body weight in ounces of water. If you weigh 160 pounds, your minimum should be 80 ounces of water. Drink one gallon if you can to clear fat, waste products, and toxins out of your body.

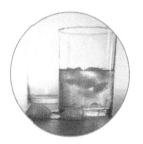

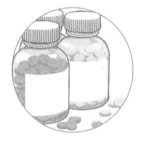

Take supplements each day. By taking the recommended supplements, you will help your body support metabolic changes, especially if you are transitioning off of prescription medication(s). Be sure to take quality supplements from reputable companies.

"We first make our habits, and then our habits make us." ~John Dryden

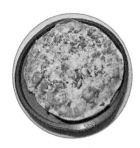

Incorporate a "treat" day once per week. While this isn't giving you a license to go hog wild on unhealthy foods, you can still have your favorite foods in balanced proportions. Treats help your metabolism to continually guess so that you never have a weight loss plateau.

Eat in front of the mirror naked. If you get off track, you may want to consider standing in your birthday suit while eating in front of the mirror. That's right! Let it be your motivation. It may be just what you need to help curb your appetite and get you back on track.

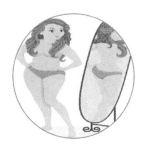

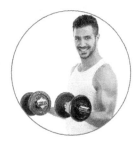

Exercise consistently. By including both aerobic and resistant exercises, you will help your basal metabolic rate and energy levels work efficiently. For best results, make sure you are consistent with your workouts. Also, allow your body to rest and heal between resistant workouts.

Add cardio exercise on an empty stomach. Work yourself up to 45 minutes of moderate intensity aerobic exercise before eating your first meal of the day. You will burn fat faster. Plus, it will give you a feeling of accomplishment and rev up your energy for the rest of the day.

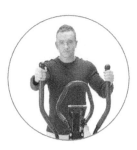

"Successful people are simply those with successful habits."
~Brain Tracy

Get quality sleep every night. Sleep 8 to 9 hours every night without interruption to help your metabolic process of losing body fat. If you can, try to put away all electronic devices like cell phones, tablets, computers, and television at least two hours before you hit the sheets as it will help you sleep better.

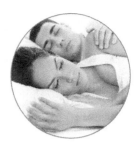

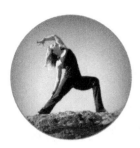

Manage stress. Avoiding drama and not getting overwhelmed over little things will help keep your cortisol levels healthy. Healthy cortisol will keep you in fat burning mode. Try yoga or meditation to help manage your stress levels.

Keep a positive mindset. Focus on your long-term goals of being fit and healthy, rather than the temporary gratification of fun or comfort foods. Add positive quotes to areas you reside throughout the day such as your desk or refrigerator. Read them each day to help you.

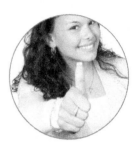

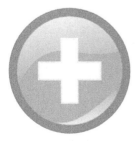

Be an example to your family, friends, and co-workers. You'll receive positive feedback if you share that you are working on being healthy, rather than telling everyone you are on a diet. Instead of being jealous of your new physique, they may just ask you for tips to start their own transformation.

"You leave old habits behind by starting out with the thought, 'I release the need for this in my life.' ~Wayne Dyer

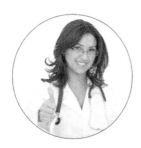

Attend regular meetings with your weight loss practitioner. If you're seeing a professional weight loss advisor, don't skip any of your assessment meetings. These encounters will help you stay on track and receive motivation which will help you to continue working towards your weight loss goals.

Live your life! Instead of focusing on food and exercise constantly, just enjoy the process and live your life. While food and exercise will help live a healthy life, but a good life will incorporate so much more. Being happy and doing the things you enjoy with your family and friends is important. Live to love!

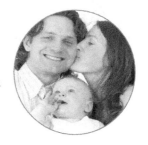

"Do what you need to do, and enjoy life as it happens."
~John Scalzi

EATING FOODS FOR GUT HEALTH & FAT LOSS

Did you know that your intestines are home to approximately 500 million bacteria? Some bacteria are good but others can be nasty. Research suggests that the more good bacteria you have in your gut, the better you are. A better gut also helps release body fat. Seems pretty straightforward.

Live microorganisms that help to restore beneficial bacteria in your gut are known as *probiotics*. Recent studies in 2015 show positive benefits to your health and gut:

- enhances immune system[54]
- suppresses malignancy of colorectal cancer cells[55/56]
- prevents and improves inflammatory bowel disease[57/58/59]
- demonstrates cholesterol-reducing potential[60]

Probiotics are essential in assisting your body with nutrient absorption. While it may not sound as nice as sipping down a delightful glass of wine, certain fermented foods can provide you with probiotics. By eating them, you naturally detoxify your body. The overall result provides you with a healthier gut which leads to fat loss and overall vitality.

If your mother insisted you eat yogurt when you had a tummy ache, there is good reason. Live-cultured yogurts have several types of probiotics in the *lactobacillus* family. Lactobacillus is a histamine producing bacteria that boosts your immunity, regulates the function of your gut, and acts as a neurotransmitter. Basically, it counteracts inflammation within the body. While yogurt may help you maintain your gut health, there are several other foods that you may want to include in your diet for gut protection. After all, your gut health is important for the health of the rest of your body. It also helps with weight loss as well.

If you have the following symptoms, you may want to include foods that will boost better gut health:

- bloating, gas, chronic diarrhea, or constipation
- excessive fatigue
- headaches
- brain fog
- memory loss
- depression or anxiety
- attention problems
- skin problems such as rash, eczema, and acne
- cravings for sugar or carbohydrates
- poor immune system
- autoimmune disease

If you have symptoms of poor gut health or trouble losing weight, you may want to include foods high in probiotics, as well as a quality probiotic supplement.

Kimchi

A popular Korean side dish, kimchi is a very spicy pickled cabbage. Aged kimchi has a plethora of probiotics as well as vitamins and calcium.[61] In 2014, the *Journal of Medicinal Food* reported kimchi's many research-proven health benefits. They include "anticancer, anti-obesity, anti-constipation, colorectal health promotion, probiotic properties, cholesterol reduction, fibrolytic effect, antioxidative and antiaging properties, brain health promotion, immune promotion, and skin health promotion.[62]

Kombucha

Used for centuries, kombucha is a sweetened black tea that has been fermented for the high amount of healthy gut probiotics it produces. A 2015 study showed that kombucha enhances biological function by enhancing antioxidant and antibacterial activities.[63] Kombucha tea may also contribute healing agents to gastric ulcers.[64] Try it hot or cold.

Microalgae

Add these superfoods to your morning routine! Microalgae plants such as blue-green algae, chlorella, and spirulina will boost probiotic protection. While microalgae aren't probiotics, they are extremely beneficial for digestion and immune health. In relation to probiotics, microalgae encourage their growth.

Pickles

Would you have thought that pickles would be a good source of probiotics? While homemade pickles are a better source than commercial brands, most have some microbial value.[65] Just be careful on your consumption of them as pickles can have a high sodium content that can lead to high blood pressure.

Sauerkraut

Traced back to the fourth century BC, sauerkraut is one of the most common and oldest forms of preserving cabbage. Made from fermented cabbage and sometimes other vegetables, sauerkraut is extremely rich in probiotics and vitamins.[66] It is also low in calories so it fits in nicely with a weight loss regimen.

Summary

Better gut health and reduced inflammation are not only great for a healthy body, but they will also help you lose body fat in record time.

KNOWING WHEN ORGANIC IS BEST

Eating the right amount of fruits and vegetables is crucial to a healthy diet. Higher consumption will help boost your immune system and ward off chronic health risks like obesity, type 2 diabetes, heart disease, cancer, and thyroid disease. However, the widespread use of pesticides in crop production comes with a range of consequences that should affect the way you think about food, including fruits and vegetables.

Ideally, pesticides sprayed on a farm field would only kill targeted pests. Unfortunately, that is not the case. Pesticides used in agriculture can contaminate the food you eat as well as the environment (air, rain, and rivers).

In a 2014 study reported in *Consumer Reports*, 89 percent of the population believes it is critical to protect the environment while 86 percent believe in the importance of reducing pesticide exposure. These statistics demonstrate an overwhelming consumer demand for foods that are healthier to the environment and consumers.

Lowering Your Exposure to Health Risks with Organic

Health risks associated with pesticides are real, but the wealth of health benefits we derive from eating fruits and vegetables is real too. A 2012 study estimated that vegetable and fruit consumption could prevent 20,000 cases of cancer per year. Another study found that people who eat vegetables and fruits at least three times per day had a lower risk of certain diseases: hypertension, heart disease, stroke, and death.

Because the benefits of vegetables and fruits are important to your health, we believe that "organic" is your best choice when consuming produce. Choosing these options can lower your personal exposure to pesticides.

High Standards of Organic Foods

Organic farmers, ranchers, and food processors must follow the United States Department of Agriculture's (USDA's) standards to grow organic food and have annual onsite inspections conducted each year. Standards cover the product from the farm to the consumer's kitchen table which includes:

- soil and water quality
- rules of food additives
- pest control
- livestock practices

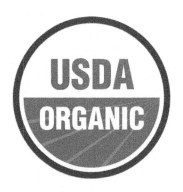

After receiving the USDA's stamp of approval, products may receive the "USDA Certified Organic" label. This label verifies that the food product has the USDA's endorsement for high standards that prohibit and restrict the use of 18 of the most potentially dangerous pesticides.[67]

Organic livestock must also be raised on certified organic land, fed 100 percent certified organic feed, and managed without the use of antibiotics, added growth hormones, and other prohibited byproducts and feed. They are also allowed year-round access to outdoors except under inclement weather.[68]

For your benefit, we are providing a list of foods that should be purchased "organic in the section below entitled "Knowing When to Buy Organic."

Peeling and Washing Away Pesticides

In a recent survey by *Consumer Reports*, about half of the population believes that peeling and washing vegetables and fruits will get rid of pesticides. While rinsing will remove the surface residues, as well as dirt and bacteria, you can't completely wash away the risk. Pesticides can stick to soft skins, and wax coatings used on certain vegetables and fruits actually trap pesticide residues. Besides, some pesticides are systemic and are taken up by the plant's root system. These pesticides can get into the flesh so that peeling and washing do nothing for it.

Even more, the USDA measures pesticide residues after the produce has already been washed and delivered to you, the consumer. Therefore, the pesticide residues used to calculate dietary risks are those that are remaining on the vegetable or fruit.

Knowing When to Buy Organic

With so many vegetables and fruits on the market, it's difficult to know which has been contaminated with pesticides. Certain agricultural crops are treated more than others, and therefore the risk for each is different. Besides, the risk is different for produce coming from different countries. Therefore, we're providing you with a list of foods that you should consider organic.

Buy Organic Vegetables - ALWAYS

- carrots
- green beans
- hot peppers
- sweet bell peppers
- sweet potatoes

Buy Organic Vegetables – RECOMMENDED

- asparagus (especially if grown in USA)
- avocado

- broccoli
- cabbage
- cauliflower
- celery (especially if grown in USA)
- cilantro
- collard greens
- corn, sweet
- cucumbers (especially if grown in Mexico or USA)
- eggplant (especially if grown in USA)
- green onions
- kale (especially if grown in USA)
- lettuce
- mushrooms
- onion
- potatoes (especially if grown in USA)
- snap peas (especially if grown in Guatemala or Peru)
- spinach
- sweet potatoes (especially if grown in USA)
- tomatoes (especially if grown in Canada, Mexico, or USA)
- summer squash (especially if grown in USA)
- winter squash (especially if grown in USA)

Buy Organic Fruits - ALWAYS

- cranberries
- nectarines
- peaches
- strawberries
- tangerines

Buy Organic Fruits - RECOMMENDED

- apples (especially if grown in USA)
- applesauce
- bananas

- blueberries
- cantaloupe (especially if grown in USA)
- cherries
- grapefruit
- grapes
- mangoes (especially if grown in Brazil)
- papaya
- peaches, canned
- pears
- pineapples
- plums (especially if grown in Chile)
- prunes or dried plums
- oranges
- raisins
- raspberries
- watermelon

Summary

Pesticides have become a nuisance. In America, the risk to the population is great because we allow them on agricultural crops. Therefore, we recommend that you check the labels and be sure to buy USDA organic produce when available – especially for the indicated foods.

TRY OUR TASTY RECIPES FOR FAT LOSS

On the following pages, you will find several delicious recipes that may help you get started on your fat loss goals. After all, your transformation process is made much simpler when you enjoy the foods you eat. So, try our recipes and keep the ones you like. Maybe they'll even spark your interest to try something new and be creative yourself. Please find our recipes and ideas on the following pages for:

- fish
- seafood
- chicken
- turkey
- egg whites
- beef & pork
- chili
- marinades
- salsas
- vegetable dips

- vegetable side dishes
- main salads
- side salads
- salad dressings
- lettuce wraps & rolls
- soups
- cereals
- snacks
- smoothies
- water and beverages

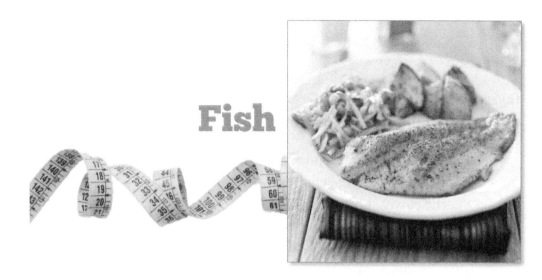

Fish

Aloha Mahi Mahi

Servings: 4

Ingredients:

- 4 4-oz. boneless Mahi Mahi fillets
- 2 cups pineapple, diced
- 1 red bell pepper, diced
- ¼ cup low-sodium chicken broth
- 2 tsp. coconut oil
- sea salt and black pepper to taste

Directions:

(1) Heat large skillet over medium-high. Cook Mahi Mahi fillets with coconut oil for about 1 minute on each side or until golden. Remove from pan and set aside.

(2) Add pineapple and bell pepper to skillet and cook for about 2 minutes or until soft. Stir in chicken broth and Mahi Mahi. Sprinkle sea salt and black pepper on top of Mahi Mahi. Cover and cook for 2 minutes. Enjoy!

Cilantro Ginger Baked Tilapia

Servings: 4

Ingredients:

- 4 5-oz. tilapia fillets
- 1 jalapeno, deseeded and chopped
- ⅓ cup cilantro leaves, chopped
- 3 garlic cloves, pressed
- 1-inch piece of ginger, minced
- 1 lemon, juiced
- 2 Tbs. Tamari sauce
- 1 tsp. sesame oil
- sea salt and black pepper to taste
- coconut oil cooking spray

Directions:

(1) Preheat oven to 450 degrees Fahrenheit.

(2) Spray 9" x 9" glass baking dish with coconut oil cooking spray.

(3) Season tilapia fillets with sea salt and black pepper. Lay fillets flat in baking dish.

(4) Place all other ingredients in a blender and puree. Pour mixture over tilapia.

(5) Bake tilapia for 30 minutes. Enjoy!

Oriental Tuna Steaks

Servings: 4

Ingredients:

- 4 5-oz. Tuna fillets
- 2 garlic cloves, pressed
- 3 Tbs. extra virgin olive oil
- 2 Tbs. Tamari sauce
- 1-½ Tbs. Dijon mustard

Directions: Mix all ingredients (except tuna) in a small mixing bowl to make a marinade for the salmon. Place tuna in a medium bakeware dish and cover with marinade. Cover dish and place in refrigerator for 1 hour. After 1 hour, remove tuna and set aside. Preheat oven to 400 degrees Fahrenheit. Place tuna in oven and bake for about 15 minutes. Enjoy!

Roasted Broccoli with Apple Salmon

Servings: 4

Ingredients:

- 4 5-oz. sockeye salmon fillets (or your choice of salmon type)
- 2 small bunches of broccoli florets, chopped
- 1 cup Vidalia onion, sliced
- 1 large sweet red apple, peeled and sliced thinly
- 3 garlic cloves, pressed
- 1 Tbs. coconut oil
- 1 lemon, juiced
- 2 tsp. Dijon mustard
- 1 cup natural apple cider
- 2 tsp. thyme flakes
- ⅛ tsp. black pepper

- ¼ tsp. red pepper flakes

Directions:

(1) Preheat oven to 400 degrees Fahrenheit.

(2) In a large pot, place broccoli. Cover with water, plus 3 to 4 inches. After water has boiled for 1 minute, remove from stovetop. Drain and rinse with cold water to stop cooking process.

(3) Transfer broccoli to a large baking dish. Add coconut oil, garlic, and red pepper flakes. Mix. Place salmon fillets on top of broccoli, and drizzle lemon juice over salmon. Rub exposed salmon with thyme and ground pepper. Bake for 10-15 minutes or until salmon is opaque and flaky.

(4) While salmon is baking, heat a large skillet over medium-high. Cook onions and apples for about 2 minutes. Stir in apple cider. Cover and reduce heat to low. Simmer for approximately 5 minutes or until onions and apples are soft. Add Dijon mustard and let cook for 2 more minutes. Add apple-onion mixture over top of salmon before serving. Enjoy!

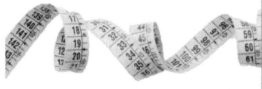

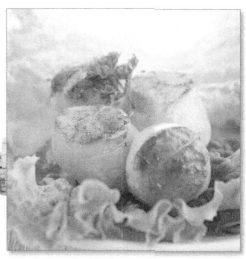

Seafood

Garlic Roasted Scallops

Servings: 4

Ingredients:

- 1 lb. scallops
- ½ cup Vidalia onion, chopped
- 3 garlic cloves, pressed
- 5 sprigs rosemary
- ¼ cup coconut oil (or coconut oil cooking spray)
- 2 Tbs. white wine vinegar
- ½ tsp. black pepper

Directions:

(1) Pour (or spray) oil into a 9" x 13" baking dish. Add rosemary, garlic, and onion. Place in oven and let sit while oven preheats to 450 degrees Fahrenheit (approximately 15 minutes).

(2) Remove baking dish from oven and add scallops and roast for approximately 4-5 minutes. Turn scallops and roast for another 4-5 minutes.

(3) Remove dish from oven and add vinegar and black pepper. Stir gently before serving. Enjoy!

Sautéed Shrimp and Broccoli

Servings: 4

Ingredients:

- 20 jumbo shrimp, peeled
- 2 small heads of broccoli florets, cut small
- 2 garlic cloves, pressed
- 1-inch piece of ginger, minced
- 1 lime, juiced
- 1 Tbs. coconut oil + 1 Tbs. coconut oil reserved
- 1 tsp. red chili peppers

Directions:

(1) Mix garlic, ginger, lime juice, and 1 Tbs. coconut oil in a large bowl. Add shrimp and mix. Place in refrigerator to marinade while preparing broccoli.

(2) Cook broccoli for 5 minutes in a vegetable steamer or microwavable dish.

(3) Heat large skillet over medium-high. Add remaining coconut oil and shrimp to sauté. Cook for approximately 5 minutes or until shrimp turns pink. Remove from pan and set aside.

(4) In same skillet, add broccoli and cook for 5 minutes. Add shrimp and cook for another minute. Remove from stovetop.

(5) Sprinkle red chili pepper flakes over shrimp before serving. Enjoy!

Chicken

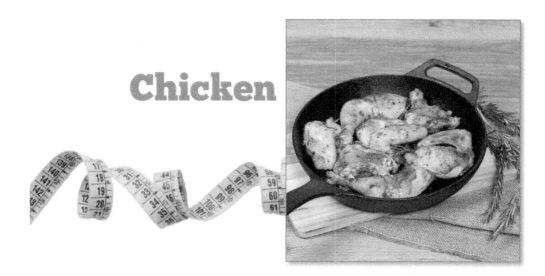

Crockpot Salsa Chicken

Servings: 4

Ingredients:

- 4 4-oz. chicken breasts, skinless and boneless
- 4 large tomatoes, diced
- ½ large onion, diced
- 1 red bell pepper, diced
- 1 cup salsa (your favorite, low-sodium)
- 1 lime, juiced
- 2 Tbs. red pepper flakes
- 1 tsp. cayenne pepper
- sea salt and black pepper to taste

Directions:

(1) Combine all ingredients except chicken in a crockpot. Mix well. Add chicken. Cook on low for about 7-8 hours.

(2) When done, shred chicken in the crockpot using a fork and knife. Mix well before serving. Enjoy!

Skillet Garlic Chicken

Servings: 4

Ingredients:

- 4 4-oz. chicken breasts or thighs
- 1 garlic clove, pressed
- 1 Tbs. coconut oil + 1 Tbs. coconut oil reserved
- 1 tsp. onion powder
- sea salt and black pepper to taste

Directions:

(1) Heat large skillet over medium-high. Turn to medium heat and add 1 Tbs. coconut oil. Sauté garlic for 1 minute.

(2) Add remaining coconut oil in skillet with chicken. Cook for approximately 8-10 minutes on each side. Sprinkle onion powder, sea salt, and black pepper while cooking.

(3) Remove from heat and serve with your favorite veggie dish!

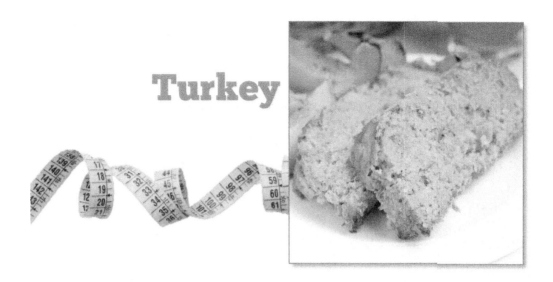

Turkey

Sweet and Spicy Turkey

Servings: 4

Ingredients for Turkey:

- 1 lb. turkey tenderloin, trimmed of visible fat
- 1 tsp. paprika
- ⅛ tsp. cayenne pepper

Ingredients for Relish:

- 2 ripe apricots, pitted and diced
- ¼ cup red onion, finely chopped
- 1 lemon, juiced (keep peel for zest)
- 1 Tbs. white wine vinegar
- 3 Tbs. fresh mint leaves

Directions:

(1) Lightly season turkey tenderloins with paprika and cayenne pepper.

(2) Heat grill or griddle. Cook turkey on medium heat for about 10 minutes on each side or until the center is no longer pink. Remove from heat and allow to cool before slicing.

(3) While turkey is cooking, combine remaining ingredients to prepare relish.

(4) Add relish on top of turkey tenderloins before serving. Enjoy!

Turkey Loaf

Servings: 4

Ingredients:

- 1 lb. ground turkey
- 1 egg
- 2 large carrots, finely chopped
- 1 large onion, finely chopped
- 1 red bell pepper, diced
- 1 stalk celery, finely chopped
- 1 garlic clove, pressed
- 1 Tbs. Worcestershire sauce
- 1 Tbs. yellow mustard
- sea salt and black pepper to taste

Directions: Preheat oven to 350 degrees Fahrenheit. Combine all ingredients and put into loaf pan. Bake for 1 hour. Enjoy!

Egg Whites

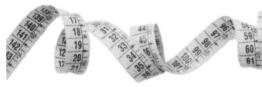

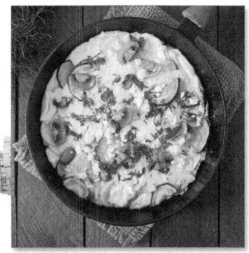

Spanish Scrambled Eggs

Servings: 2

Ingredients:

- 6 egg whites
- 2 whole Omega-3 eggs
- 2 zucchinis, julienned
- 2 Roma tomatoes, diced
- 2 red bell peppers, diced
- 1 onion, chopped
- 1 Tbs. coconut oil
- ½ tsp. oregano
- ½ tsp. paprika
- sea salt and black pepper to taste

Directions: In a large bowl, whisk egg whites, oregano, paprika, sea salt, and black pepper. Set aside. Heat large skillet on high. Add coconut oil and sauté all vegetables for approximately 3 minutes or until soft. Drizzle eggs over top and continue cooking and stirring until egg whites are cooked through.

Zucchini Frittata

Servings: 2

Ingredients:

- 6 egg whites
- 2 whole Omega-3 eggs
- 2 cups zucchini, diced
- 1 small Vidalia onion, chopped
- ½ cup shiitake mushroom, sliced
- ¼ cup parsley, chopped
- 1 garlic clove, pressed
- 1 Tbs. coconut oil

Directions: In a large bowl, combine all ingredients (except oil) and mix well. Heat oil in a large skillet over medium-high. Add egg mixture and cook until golden brown on bottom. Then flip and cook other side until golden. Cut into wedges before serving.

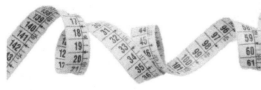

Beef & Pork

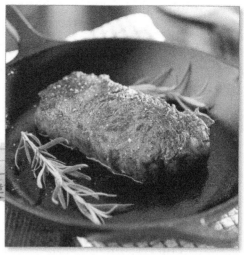

Mixed Mushroom Steak

Servings: 4

Ingredients:

- 4 5-oz. top sirloin steaks, trimmed of visible fat
- 1 lb. Portobello mushrooms (or your desired mushrooms), sliced
- 3 garlic cloves, pressed
- ½ cup low-sodium beef broth
- 1 Tbs. Worcestershire sauce
- 1 Tbs. coconut oil
- 1 Tbs. thyme flakes
- sea salt and black pepper to taste

Directions:

(1) Heat large skillet, and add coconut oil and steaks to cook over medium-high heat. Season steaks with sea salt and black pepper. Cook for 4 minutes per side or desired wellness. Remove from skillet and set aside.

(2) Add garlic to skillet and cook for 1 minute. Add mushrooms, broth, thyme, and Worcestershire sauce. Cook and stir for 3-5 minutes. Place mushrooms over steak before serving. Enjoy!

Pear Spiced Pork Tenderloins

Servings: 4

Ingredients:

- 1 pound pork tenderloin
- 1 large pear, firm and diced
- ¼ cup red onion, chopped
- ½ lemon, juiced & 2 tsp. lemon rind, grated
- 2-inch piece of ginger, minced
- 1 tsp. coconut oil
- ½ tsp. each of cinnamon & cumin
- sea salt and black pepper to taste

Directions:

(1) Preheat oven to 425 degrees Fahrenheit.

(2) Combine pear, onion, ginger, lemon juice, and lemon zest in a small bowl. Mix and set aside.

(3) Brush coconut oil over pork. Combine cinnamon, cumin, cayenne, sea salt, and black pepper in another small bowl. Mix and sprinkle mixture evenly over pork.

(4) Heat skillet and brown pork over medium-high for 4 minutes on each side. Transfer pork to baking sheet and bake for 20 minutes or until barely pink in the center. Remove pork from oven and let cool for 5 minutes. Slice thin and place on plate. Add pear mixture over pork tenderloin before serving. Enjoy!

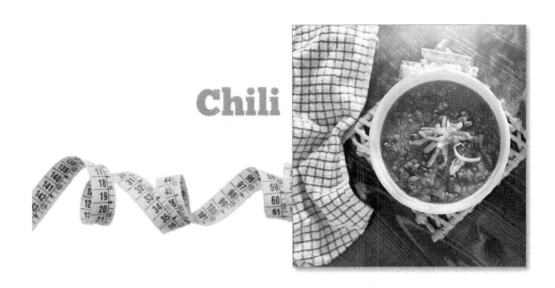

Chili

Beef & Bean Chili

Servings: 8

Ingredients:

- 1 lb. ground beef, lean
- 1 medium onion, chopped
- 1 green bell pepper, chopped
- 2 garlic cloves, pressed
- 2 8-oz. cans tomato sauce, organic, no salt added
- 1 14-16 oz. can kidney beans, rinsed and drained
- 1 14-16 oz. can great northern beans, rinsed and drained
- 1 14-16 oz. can garbanzo beans, rinsed and drained
- 1 14-16 oz. can black beans, rinsed and drained
- 1 Tbs. coconut oil
- 1-¾ cups purified water
- 2-½ tsp. hot sauce
- 1 Tbs. cocoa powder
- 1 tsp. chili powder
- ½ tsp. cayenne pepper
- ½ tsp. black pepper

- ½ cup Greek yogurt
- ½ cup cheddar cheese, shredded

Directions:

(1) Heat large pot, and add coconut oil over medium. Cook beef, onions, pepper, and garlic. Cook until meat is no longer pink. Drain excess fat.

(2) Stir in water, tomato sauce, beans, hot sauce, cocoa, and seasonings. Bring to a boil. Reduce heat. Cover and simmer for 30 minutes, stirring occasionally.

(3) Garnish each serving with 1 Tbs. of Greek yogurt and 1 Tbs. of cheddar cheese. Serve and enjoy!

Christmas Chili

Servings: 4

Ingredients:

- 1 lb. chicken breasts, boneless & skinless, but into bite size
- 1 Tbs. olive oil
- 1 (14-16 oz.) can Cannellini or Great Northern beans
- 1 (14-16 oz.) can light red kidney beans
- 1 small onion, finely chopped
- 1 cup water
- 2 cloves garlic, pressed
- 2 Tbs. chili powder
- 1 Tbs. basil, dried
- 4 cups spinach, fresh

Directions:

(1) Heat medium-sized pot on stovetop on medium-high heat. Add olive oil, onions, garlic, and chicken. Cook through. Add beans,

water, and spices and mix well. Bring to a boil. Reduce heat and simmer for 20 minutes.

(2) Add spinach and cook for two more minutes while stirring lightly.

(3) Remove from heat and serve. Enjoy!

Turkey Vegetable Chili

Servings: 4

Ingredients:

- 1 lb. ground turkey, lean
- 8 oz. canned black beans, rinsed and drained
- 4 cups baby spinach
- 4 medium tomatoes, diced
- 1 yellow bell pepper, diced
- 1 large celery stalk, diced
- 1 large carrot, peeled and diced
- 1 large onion, diced
- 1 red chili pepper, seeded and diced small
- 2 garlic cloves, pressed
- ½ Tbs. coconut oil + 1 Tbs. coconut oil reserved
- ¼ cup plain Greek yogurt
- 1 tsp. cumin
- sea salt and black pepper to taste
- fresh chives to garnish

Directions:

(1) Heat small pot and drizzle ½ Tbs. coconut oil over medium-high. Add ground turkey. Stir occasionally until turkey is cooked through. Drain any excess fat and set aside.

(2) Heat large pot and drizzle remaining 1 Tbs. coconut oil over medium-high.

(3) Add onions, red chili peppers, and garlic. Sauté for 2 minutes or until tender.

(4) Sprinkle cumin over onion mixture and stir well.

(5) Add celery, carrot, and bell pepper. Cook for 5 minutes, stirring occasionally or until vegetables begin to tenderize.

(6) Add tomatoes and beans. Cook for 8 minutes, stirring occasionally or until tomatoes have broken down and most of the liquid has evaporated.

(7) Stir in spinach until slightly wilted.

(8) Add cooked turkey and mix through. Remove from heat.

(9) Season the chili to taste with sea salt and black pepper.

(10) Spoon the chili onto serving dishes and spoon 1 Tbs. of Greek yogurt onto each of the 4 bowls. Garnish with chives and serve. Enjoy!

Marinades

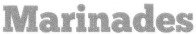
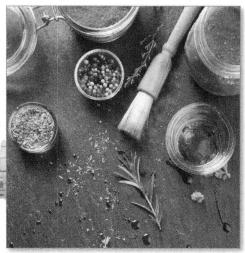
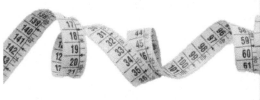

Mix all recipe ingredients for marinades in airtight jars and keep in the refrigerator. Marinade your meats overnight or a few hours for best taste. This allows the flavors to soak into the meats. Be creative and try mixing your own marinades too!

Chicken Marinade

- 1-½ cup extra virgin olive oil
- ¾ cup tamari sauce
- 1/3 cup Worcestershire sauce
- ½ cup red wine vinegar
- 1/3 cup lemon juice
- 2 Tbs. dry mustard
- 1 tsp. sea salt
- 1 Tbs. black pepper
- 1-½ tsp. fresh parsley

Fish Marinade

- ¼ cup extra virgin olive oil
- 1/3 cup lemon juice
- 1 lime, juiced

- 3 garlic cloves, minced
- 4 tsp. paprika
- 2 tsp. cumin
- 1 tsp. sea salt & black pepper
- 1-½ Tbs. parsley, ground
- 1-½ Tbs. coriander, ground

Pork Tenderloin Marinade

- ¼ cup extra virgin olive oil
- ¼ cup tamari sauce
- 3 Tbs. Dijon honey mustard
- 1 garlic clove, mined
- pinch of sea salt & black pepper

Poultry Marinade

- ¼ cup water
- ¼ cup tamari sauce
- 1 tsp. Sirachi sauce (optional)
- ¾ cup lemon juice
- ¼ tsp. Stevia, granulated or raw
- ¼ tsp. onion powder
- ¼ tsp. ginger, ground

Steak Marinade

- ½ cup extra virgin olive oil
- ¼ cup tamari sauce
- 2-½ Tbs. red wine vinegar
- 2 Tbs. lemon juice
- 1 Tbs. Dijon mustard
- ½ onion, finely chopped
- 1 garlic clove, minced
- 1 ½ Tbs. black pepper

Salsas

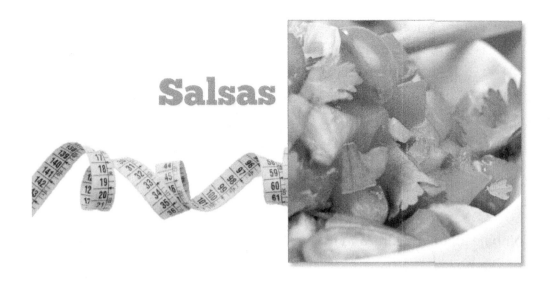

Avocado Salsa

Combine all ingredients and toss well. Refrigerate for 1 hour before serving. Enjoy!

Ingredients:

- 1 avocado, peeled and diced
- 2 Roma tomatoes, chopped
- 1 small onion, chopped
- 1 garlic clove, pressed
- ½ lemon, juice
- 1 Tbs. extra virgin olive oil
- sea salt and black pepper to taste

Black Bean Garden Salsa

Combine all ingredients and toss well. If allowed to sit for a few hours, the ingredients will infuse together for better flavor.

Ingredients:

- 1-¼ cup black beans
- 2 tomatoes, diced

- 1 onion, diced finely
- 1-½ cup fresh cilantro, chopped
- 1½ Tbs. garlic, minced
- 1-½ tsp. cayenne pepper
- ½ Tbs. hemp oil
- ½ Tbs. flaxseed oil
- 2 lime, cut into small pieces

Mama's Homemade Salsa

Combine all ingredients and toss well. Refrigerate for 1 hour before serving. Enjoy!

Ingredients:

- 3 large ripe tomatoes, seeds removed and chopped
- ¼ cup sweet onion, finely chopped
- 1 large hot chili pepper (jalapeno or Serrano)
- 2 small cloves garlic, pressed
- 2-3 Tbs. fresh cilantro, chopped
- 1-½ Tbs. lime juice
- Sea salt and black pepper to taste

Mango Pepper Salsa

Combine all ingredients and toss well. Refrigerate for 1 hour before serving. Enjoy!

Ingredients:

- 4 red bell peppers, chopped
- 2 large ripe mangos, diced
- 2 scallions, sliced
- 1 jalapeno, chopped finely
- 1 bunch cilantro, finely chopped
- ½ lime, juice

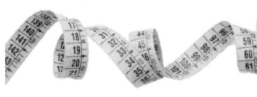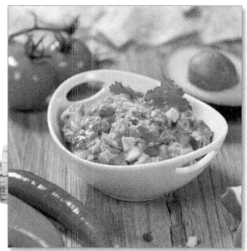

Black Bean Hummus

Add all ingredients (except olive oil) to a food processor. Puree until smooth. Add olive oil as needed to thin. Enjoy!

Ingredients:

- 1 15-oz. can black beans, drained and rinsed
- ½ cup fresh cilantro, chopped fine
- 1 garlic clove, pressed
- extra virgin olive oil (as needed for thinning)
- 2 Tbs. lemon juice
- 2 Tbs. tahini
- ½ tsp. cumin
- ½ tsp. cayenne pepper
- ½ tsp. paprika
- ½ tsp. sea salt

Guacamole

Mix all ingredients until combined well. Don't overmix. Enjoy!

Ingredients:

- 3 avocados, ripe
- ½ red onion, minced well
- 1 jalapeno, chopped finely
- 1 garlic clove, pressed
- 2 Tbs. cilantro, chopped finely
- ½ lime, juiced

Raw Chickpea-Less Hummus

Mix all ingredients until combined well. Enjoy!

Ingredients:

- 2 zucchinis, peeled and chopped
- 3 garlic cloves, pressed
- 2 Tbs. nutritional yeast
- ¾ cup tahini
- 2 tsp. sea salt

Red Pepper Hummus

Mix all ingredients in a food processor and blend until smooth. Enjoy!

- ½ roasted red bell pepper
- 1 can (15 oz.) garbanzo beans
- 2 Tbs. lemon juice
- 1 Tbs. extra virgin olive oil
- 1 Tbs. garlic, pressed
- 1 Tbs. sesame seeds
- 1 tsp. black pepper

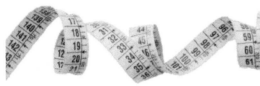

Veggie Sides

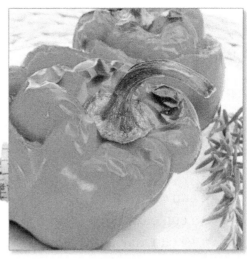

Crispy Kale Chips

Serves: 4

Ingredients:

- 4 cups kale, stalks removed and chopped
- 1 Tbs. olive oil
- ¼ cup almonds, sliced
- Seasoning of your choice (garlic powder, sea salt, ground pepper, paprika, rosemary, etc.)

Directions:

(1) Preheat oven to 275 degrees Fahrenheit.

(2) In a medium mixing bowl, toss kale leaves with olive oil, almonds, and seasoning. Lay mixture flat on baking sheet. Bake for about 15-20 minutes (or until leaves are crispy). Turn leaves halfway through.

Eggplant Parmigiana

Servings: 4

Ingredients:

- 1 large eggplant, sliced
- 1-½ cup kale, minced
- 1/3 cup almond flour
- 1 cup egg whites
- ½ cup olive oil
- 1 ½ cup marinara sauce
- 1 tomato, finely diced
- 1 clove garlic, pressed
- 2 cups mozzarella cheese
- ½ cup parmesan cheese
- Ground pepper to taste

Directions:

(1) Preheat oven to 375 degrees Fahrenheit.

(2) In a small bowl, add flour. In another small bowl, and egg whites.

(3) Lightly coat eggplant with flour by dipping into bowl. Then dip the floured eggplant into egg whites.

(4) Heat large skillet on medium. Add olive oil and let get hot. Add dipped eggplant. Sauté for about 10 minutes (5 minutes on each side). Continue until all slices are sautéed.

(5) In a baking dish, add ½ cup of marinara sauce to bottom. Add layers in order:

   a. Sautéed eggplant
   b. Kale
   c. Diced tomato

d. Mozzarella

Repeat layers with remaining ingredients. Add the remaining marina sauce to top. Then add parmesan cheese and ground pepper to the top. Bake for 20 minutes. Serve and enjoy!

Lemon Roasted Peppers

Servings: 4

Ingredients:

- 2 red bell peppers, sliced
- 1 yellow bell pepper, sliced
- 1 orange bell pepper, sliced
- 2 green bell peppers, sliced
- 5 small sweet peppers (any color), chopped
- 1 lemon, juiced
- ½ tsp. coconut oil
- sea salt and pepper to taste

Directions: Set oven to broil. Place peppers on baking sheet. Coat peppers with coconut oil, and broil for 2-3 minutes or until skin is browned. Drizzle lemon juice and sprinkle sea salt and black pepper over vegetables before serving. Enjoy!

Roasted Florets and Peppers

Servings: 4

Ingredients:

- 1 head broccoli florets, chopped to bite size
- 1 head cauliflower florets, chopped to bit size
- 1 red bell pepper, sliced
- 1 orange or yellow bell pepper, sliced
- 1 green bell pepper, sliced

- ½ medium Vidalia onion, chopped
- 3 Tbs. coconut oil
- ¾ tsp. red pepper flakes
- sea salt and black pepper to taste

Directions: Preheat oven to 400 degrees Fahrenheit. Lay vegetables on a large baking dish. Drizzle coconut oil and sprinkle spices over vegetables. Roast for about 10 minutes. Flip vegetables and roast for another 10 minutes. Remove from oven and serve. Enjoy!

Zucchini Fries

Serves: 4

Ingredients:

- 4 small zucchini, trimmed and cut into "fries"
- 1 Tbs. extra virgin olive oil
- 1 tsp. garlic, pressed
- ½ tsp. sea salt & ½ tsp. black pepper
- 2 Tbs. Parmigiano-Reggiano cheese, finely grated

Directions:

(1) Preheat oven to 450 degrees Fahrenheit.

(2) Line a rimmed baking sheet with foil and coat with cooking spray.

(3) In a large mixing bowl, combine zucchini, oil, garlic, salt, and pepper. Toss to coat thoroughly.

(4) Arrange zucchini on prepared baking sheet in a single layer and roast. Bake for 18 to 20 minutes or until tender and lightly browned. Toss halfway through cooking.

(5) Transfer to plate. Sprinkle cheese and serve. Enjoy!

Main Salads

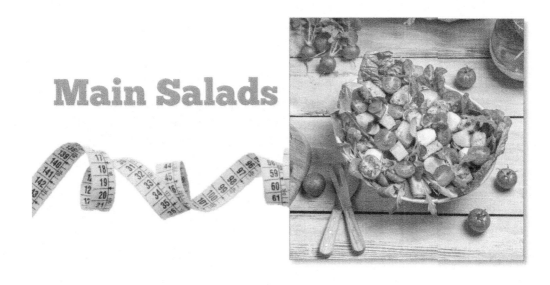

Sweet Halibut Salad

Servings: 4

Ingredients:

- 4 6-oz. halibut steaks, skinless and bones removed
- 6 cups baby spinach
- ½ cup cucumber, peeled and diced
- 3 cups strawberries, sliced
- 2 kiwis, peeled and diced
- ½ lemon, juiced
- 1 Tbs. extra virgin olive oil
- ¼ tsp. cayenne pepper
- ¼ tsp. cinnamon
- black pepper to taste

Directions:

(1) In a medium bowl, mix spices to make a rub for fish. Gently rub spices into halibut.

(2) Heat large skillet (or electric skillet) on medium-high. Cook halibut for approximately 4 minutes on each side or until opaque and flaky.

(3) While fish is cooking, make a salad mixture by combining spinach, cucumber, strawberries, kiwis, lemon juice, and olive oil. Mix well.

(4) Top salad mixture with halibut before serving. Enjoy!

Tasty Tuna Salad

Servings: 1

Ingredients:

- 3-oz. can solid white tuna, drained and shredded
- ½ head of Butter lettuce, torn into bite-sized pieces
- 8 grape tomatoes
- 1 stalk celery, chopped
- ½ orange bell pepper, chopped
- ½ small Vidalia onion, chopped
- ¼ tsp. garlic powder
- 1 Tbs. extra virgin olive oil

Directions: Combine all ingredients and let marinade in refrigerator for 1 hour before serving. Enjoy!

Tropical Chicken Salad

Servings: 4

Ingredients:

- 1 lbs. chicken breast, cooked and diced
- 1 large bag pre-washed mixed greens
- ½ lime, juiced
- ¼ cup Greek yogurt, plain

- 1 (7-8 oz. can) tropical fruit, unsweetened and drained
- 1 tsp. curry powder

Directions:

(1) In a small bowl, add yogurt, lime juice, and curry powder. Mix well and set aside.

(2) In a medium bowl, add chicken, tropical fruit, and contents from small bowl. Mix well to coat chicken and fruit.

(3) Divide mixed greens between 4 plates and top each with chicken salad. Serve and enjoy!

Warm Spinach Chicken Salad

Servings: 4

Ingredients:

- 1 lb. chicken breast, diced
- 1 14-oz. package of organic spinach leaves
- 2 medium tomatoes, diced
- 2 garlic cloves, pressed
- 1 Tbs. coconut oil + 1 Tbs. coconut oil reserved
- sea salt and black pepper to taste

Directions:

(1) Heat medium sauce pan, and add 1 Tbs. coconut oil and garlic. Cook for 30 seconds.

(2) Add spinach and cover. Cook 1-3 minutes until leaves begin to wilt. Uncover and stir spinach. Cover and cook another 3-5 minutes or until leaves are completely wilted.

(3) Remove spinach from heat and place in a large bowl. Set aside. Add remaining coconut oil to sauce pan with chicken. Sprinkle

sea salt and black pepper. Cook until done, stirring occasionally. Remove from heat and add to top spinach. Add diced tomatoes to top spinach and chicken. Serve and enjoy!

Yum-Yum Salad

Servings: 4

Ingredients:

- 1 lb. lean turkey or chicken sausage, sliced
- 3 cups apples, diced
- 7 cups fresh spinach
- ½ cup quinoa, cooked
- ½ cup walnuts, crushed

Directions:

(1) In a medium skillet, sauté sausage until cooked through and lightly browned. Set aside to cool.

(2) Combine all ingredients in a large mixing bowl.

(3) Drizzle your favorite salad dressing and mix well. Serve and enjoy!

Side Salads

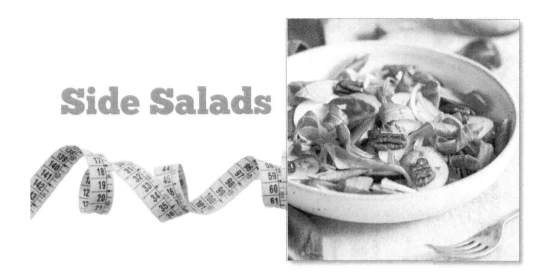

Artichoke Salad

Servings: 4

Ingredients:

- ➢ 1 head Romaine lettuce, cut into wedges
- ➢ 3 artichoke hearts, cut into wedges
- ➢ 1 red bell pepper, sliced thin
- ➢ 1 cucumber, peeled and sliced
- ➢ 3 garlic cloves, pressed
- ➢ 2 tsp. extra virgin olive oil
- ➢ 2 tsp. Dijon mustard
- ➢ 1 Tbs. white wine vinegar
- ➢ sea salt and black pepper to taste

Directions: In a large bowl, make salad mixture by combining lettuce, artichoke, bell pepper, and cucumber. In a small bowl, make a dressing by whisking together the garlic, olive oil, mustard, vinegar, sea salt, and black pepper. Drizzle with dressing before serving. Enjoy!

Avocado Walnut Salad

Servings: 4

Ingredients:

- ➢ 1 head Romaine lettuce, torn into small pieces
- ➢ 3 avocados, peeled and sliced
- ➢ 1 tsp. lemon juice
- ➢ ¼ cup walnuts, chopped
- ➢ 3 Tbs. extra virgin olive oil
- ➢ 2 Tbs. red wine vinegar

Directions: In a large bowl, mix all ingredients (except olive oil and vinegar) to prepare salad mixture. In a small bowl, whisk olive oil and vinegar to prepare dressing. Drizzle over salad mixture and serve. Enjoy!

Pear and Toasted Walnut Salad

Servings: 4

Ingredients:

- 6 cups baby arugula leaves
- 2 pears, thinly sliced
- 1 ½ Tbs. shallots, minced
- ¼ cup walnuts, chopped and toasted
- 2 Tbs. extra virgin olive oil
- 2 Tbs. white wine vinegar
- ¼ tsp. Dijon mustard
- ¼ tsp. black pepper

Directions: In a large bowl, combine shallots, olive oil, vinegar, mustard, and black pepper. Stir with a whisk. Add arugula and pears to bowl and coat well. Serve mixture to 4 plates. Spring each serving with 1 Tbs. walnuts. Enjoy!

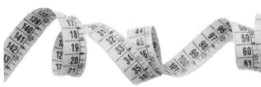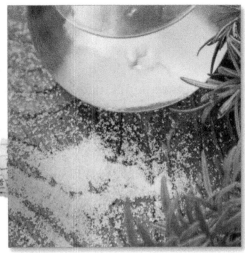

Dressings

Basil Nut Vinaigrette

Blend all ingredients (except walnuts) until smooth. Stir in walnuts. Chill before serving. Enjoy!

- 20 fresh basil leaves, chopped fine
- 1 garlic clove, pressed
- 2 Tbs. extra virgin olive oil
- 2 Tbs. wine vinegar
- 2 tsp. Dijon mustard
- 4 Tbs. low-sodium chicken broth
- 2 Tbs. walnuts, chopped
- sea salt and black pepper to taste

Caesar Dressing

Blend all ingredients together until smooth. Chill before serving. Enjoy!

- 1 garlic clove, pressed
- 1 Tbs. lemon juice
- 2 Tbs. extra virgin olive oil
- 1 tsp. dry mustard
- 1 tsp. cayenne pepper

- sea salt and black pepper to taste

Garlic Dressing

Blend all ingredients together until smooth. Chill before serving. Enjoy!

- 2 garlic cloves, pressed
- 3 Tbs. virgin olive oil
- 1 Tbs. tarragon vinegar
- 2 Tbs. lemon juice
- ½ tsp. dry mustard
- 1 tsp. black pepper

Granny Apple Vinaigrette

Add all ingredients to a blender and puree. Chill before serving. Enjoy!

- 1 Gala apple, peeled and chopped
- ½ cup walnut oil
- ¼ cup apple cider vinegar
- ½ tsp. paprika
- ½ tsp. cinnamon
- ½ tsp. red pepper flakes

Red Wine Vinaigrette

Combine all ingredients together until smooth. Chill before serving. Enjoy!

- 2 garlic cloves, pressed
- ½ cup fresh basil leaves, chopped fine
- ½ cup fresh parsley, chopped fine
- 1 cup extra virgin olive oil
- ½ cup red wine vinegar
- 2 Tbs. Dijon mustard
- 1 tsp. black pepper

Wraps & Rolls

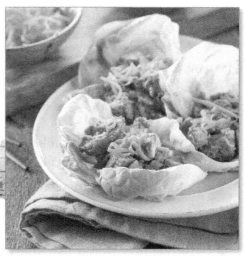

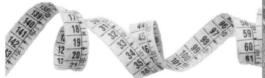

Chicken Lettuce Tacos

Servings: 4

Ingredients:

- 1 lb. ground chicken breast
- 1 large head of Romaine lettuce leaves
- 2 tomatoes, chopped
- 1 green bell pepper, chopped
- ½ onion, chopped
- 1 jalapeno pepper, deseeded and chopped (optional)
- 1 Tbs. lime juice
- 1 Tbs. coconut oil

Directions: Heat a large skillet, and cook coconut oil and chicken on medium-high. Stir occasionally until chicken is cooked through. While chicken is cooking, mix vegetables (except lettuce) and add lime juice. Spoon chicken and vegetable mixture into lettuce leaves to make wrap. Enjoy!

Steak Lettuce Wrap

Servings: 4

Ingredients:

- 1 lb. sirloin steak, boneless and trimmed of visible fat
- 1 large head of butter lettuce
- 1 medium carrot, peeled and sliced thin
- ½ cup red onion, sliced thin
- ½ cucumber, peeled and sliced thin
- 1 cup cherry tomatoes, quartered
- 2 garlic cloves, pressed
- 1 Tbs. coconut oil
- 1 Tbs. balsamic vinegar
- 3 Tbs. Dijon mustard
- ¾ tsp. red pepper flakes

Directions: Marinate steaks in vinegar for about 10 minutes. While steak is marinating, prepare lettuce leaves by topping with carrots, onions, cucumbers, and tomatoes. Heat large skillet, and cook oil and garlic for 1 minute over medium-high. Add steak and cook for 4 minutes on each side. Remove and let cool slightly. Cut into thin strips and top lettuce wraps. Add mustard and red pepper flakes to each wrap before serving. Enjoy!

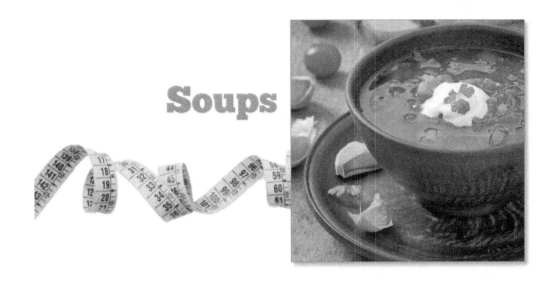

Soups

Avocado Scallop Soup

Servings: 4

Ingredients:

- 1 lb. small bay scallops
- 2 cups plum tomatoes, chopped
- 1 cup cucumber, peeled, seeded, and chopped
- ¾ cup roasted red pepper, chopped
- ½ cup scallions, chopped
- ⅓ cup celery, chopped
- ½ avocado + ½ avocado reserved and sliced
- ¾ cup low-sodium tomato juice
- 2 Tbs. lemon, juiced
- 1-½ Tbs. dried cilantro
- ½ Tbs. dried parsley
- 1 Tbs. red wine vinegar
- 2 Tbs. coconut oil
- ¼ tsp. sea salt + ¼ tsp. sea salt reserved
- ¼ tsp. black pepper + ¼ tsp. black pepper reserved

Directions:

(1) Add to blender: tomatoes, cucumber, red pepper, scallions, celery, ½ avocado, scallions, tomato juice, lemon juice, cilantro, parsley, vinegar, sea salt, and black pepper. Blend until desired consistency is reached. Cover and chill in refrigerator for at least 1 hour or overnight to let flavors meld.

(2) When ready to serve, pat scallops dry and season with remaining sea salt and black pepper.

(3) Heat skillet and add coconut oil over medium-high. Add scallops and sear for approximately 2 minutes per side (or to desired doneness). Scallops should be ready when they are no longer translucent.

(4) Divide gazpacho (cold soup) between 4 bowls. Top with scallops and avocado slices. Serve and enjoy!

Spicy Ginger Soup

Servings: 4

Ingredients:

- 1 lb. shrimp, peeled (can use chicken, turkey, or beef if desired)
- 4 cups low-sodium vegetable broth
- ½ cup celery, chopped
- ½ cup carrots, chopped
- ½ cup onions, chopped
- ½ cup snow peas
- 2-inch piece of ginger, unpeeled
- 3 garlic cloves, pressed
- 1 Thai chili pepper, chopped in half (seeds removed if desired)
- ½ cup cilantro, chopped finely
- sea salt and black pepper to taste

Directions:

(1) Heat large pot on high. Add broth. When broth is hot, add cilantro, ginger, garlic, chili pepper, sea salt, and black pepper. When broth comes to a boil, turn heat to medium and simmer for 5 minutes.

(2) Strain broth into another bowl. Remove remaining ingredients from pot and throw away. Return strained broth to pot. Add vegetables and simmer for 20-30 minutes.

(3) Add shrimp and cook for 5 minutes or until shrimp is pink. Remove from heat and serve. Enjoy!

Spicy Kale Chowder with Sausage

Servings: 12

Ingredients:

- 1 lb. low-fat spicy turkey or chicken sausage, sliced ¼-inch thick
- 1 bunch kale, destalked and chopped
- 2 large onions, chopped
- 1 28-oz. can organic Italian plum tomatoes, chopped with juices reserved
- 8 garlic cloves, minced
- 2 Tbs. ginger, minced
- 3 qt. low-sodium turkey or chicken broth
- sea salt and black pepper to taste
- coconut oil cooking spray

Directions: Heat large cooking pot over medium-high. Spray coconut oil in bottom of the pot, and add garlic and onions; stir occasionally until soft – about 10 minutes. Add sausage and ginger and cook for 5 minutes while stirring occasionally. Add the tomatoes and juices. Bring to a boil. Add the stock and kale and return to boil. Reduce heat to medium, and simmer until kale is tender – about 10 minutes. Season with sea salt and black pepper. Enjoy!

Tofu and Chicken Soup

Servings: 4

Ingredients:

- 1-½ cups chicken breast, shredded
- 14 oz. package of extra firm tofu, cubed
- ¼ cup egg whites
- 3-½ cups low-sodium chicken broth
- 1 cup cabbage, cooked and shredded (can use coleslaw mix)
- 3-4 garlic cloves, minced
- 1 Tbs. coconut oil
- 3 Tbs. rice vinegar
- 2 Tbs. Tamari sauce
- 1 tsp. sesame oil
- ½ tsp. crushed red pepper flakes
- sea salt and black pepper to taste

Directions:

(1) Heat a large pot, and add coconut oil and garlic over medium heat and sauté for 1 minute. Add broth, vinegar, Tamari sauce, and red pepper flakes. Bring to a boil.

(2) Add chicken and tofu. Lower heat and simmer for 10 minutes.

(3) Add egg whites, stirring to mix.

(4) Add cabbage and simmer for another 5 minutes. Remove from heat.

(5) Stir in sesame oil.

(6) Serve and enjoy!

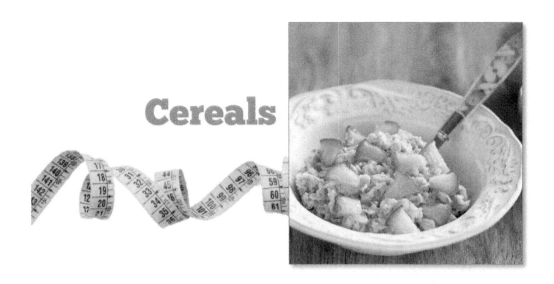

Cereals

Granny's Apple Oatmeal

Servings: 4

Ingredients:

- 2 cups Old Fashioned oats
- 2 Tbs. protein powder, vanilla
- ½ Tbs. slivered almonds
- ½ cup craisins
- 1 large apple, grated
- 2 cups pure unsweetened almond milk
- 4 Tbs. maple syrup, 100% grade A or B
- ½ tsp. vanilla extract
- 1-½ tsp. cinnamon
- coconut oil cooking spray

Directions: Preheat oven to 400 degrees Fahrenheit. Spray a large (3-quart) baking dish with coconut oil cooking spray. In a large bowl, combine all ingredients and mix well. Pour mixture into baking dish and bake uncovered for 45 minutes. Enjoy!

Quinoa Cinnamon Porridge

Servings: 4

Ingredients:

- ½ cup quinoa, uncooked
- 1 large apple, diced
- ½ cup blueberries
- ½ cup pure unsweetened almond milk
- 1 cup purified water
- 1 tsp. vanilla extract
- 2 Tbs. walnuts or pecans, chopped
- 1-½ tsp. cinnamon
- 1-2 packets of Stevia (optional)

Directions: Add quinoa, water, and cinnamon to a small cooking pot and bring to a boil over high heat. Reduce heat to low. Cover and simmer for 15 minutes or until most of the water has been absorbed. Uncover, add almond milk, and simmer for an additional 10 minutes. Stir in apples, blueberries, vanilla extract, and nuts. Cover and let sit for 10 minutes before serving. Porridge will thicken during this time. If desired, add Stevia to sweeten porridge. Enjoy!

Snacks

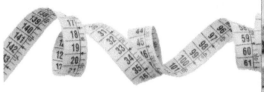
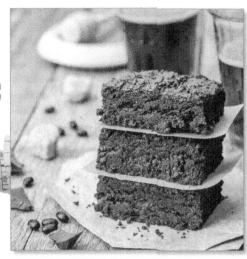

Apple Crisp

Servings: 2

Ingredients:

- 2 small Gala apples, sliced
- ¼ cup Old Fashioned oats
- 1 Tbs. cinnamon
- ½ tsp. nutmeg
- 2 packets Stevia
- coconut oil cooking spray

Directions:

(1) Preheat oven to 350 degrees Fahrenheit.

(2) Arrange apple slices in baking pan, coated with coconut oil cooking spray.

(3) Mix remaining ingredients and sprinkle over apples.

(4) Bake for 30-35 minutes or until topping is golden brown and apples are tender. Enjoy!

Bake-Free Chocolate Oatmeal Bars

Servings: 9

Ingredients:

- 1-½ cup Old Fashioned oats
- 2 scoops whey protein powder, chocolate
- 1 cup fat-free powdered milk
- ½ cup craisins or raisins
- ¼ cup pure peanut butter
- ¼ cup purified water
- 2 tsp. vanilla extract
- 2 Tbs. flaxseeds
- 1 Tbs. cinnamon
- coconut oil cooking spray

Directions:

(1) Lightly spray an 8-inch square pan with coconut oil cooking spray.

(2) In a large mixing bowl, combine oats, whey, powdered milk, and cinnamon. Mix well and set aside.

(3) In a medium mixing bowl, whisk together peanut butter, water, and vanilla extract. Add the peanut butter mixture to the oat mixture in the large bowl. Stir to form sticky dough. Add raisins and knead evenly.

(4) Using wet hands or a spatula, spread the mixture evenly into 8-inch square pan. Freeze for 1 hour or refrigerate overnight.

(5) When mixture is firm to cut, cut into 9 squares. Serve or wrap individually and store in refrigerator. Enjoy!

Chocolate Walnut Pudding

Servings: 4

Ingredients:

- 2 scoops protein powder, chocolate
- 4 tsp. unsweetened cocoa powder
- ¼ cup walnuts, chopped
- 1 pint plain Greek yogurt
- 4 cups raspberries
- 2 packets Stevia

Directions:

(1) Combine all ingredients (except raspberries and walnuts). Mix well.

(2) Portion out mixture into 4 dessert bowls.

(3) Top each bowl with ¼ cup raspberries and 1 Tbs. walnuts before serving. Enjoy!

Guilt-Free Brownies

Servings: 16

Ingredients:

- 1 14-16 oz. can black beans, rinsed and drained
- 12 oz. package extra-firm tofu
- 3 whole Omega-3 eggs
- ½ cup unsweetened applesauce
- 2 Tbs. coconut oil
- ⅓ cup maple syrup, 100% pure
- 2 tsp. vanilla extract
- ¾ cup protein powder, chocolate
- ½ cup unsweetened cocoa powder

- 1 tsp. baking powder
- 1 Tbs. cinnamon
- coconut oil cooking spray

Directions:

(1) Preheat oven to 350 degrees Fahrenheit.

(2) Puree beans in food processor. Add the rest of the wet ingredients and blend to combine (tofu, eggs, applesauce, coconut oil, maple syrup, and vanilla extract). Set aside.

(3) In a large mixing bowl, use a fork to mix together dry ingredients (protein powder, cocoa powder, baking powder, and cinnamon).

(4) Add wet ingredients to dry ingredients in large mixing bowl. Blend until creamy smooth.

(5) Spray an 8" x 8" baking dish with coconut oil cooking spray. Bake for 30 minutes or until a knife inserted comes out clean. Serve and enjoy!

Nutty Chocolate Squares

Serves: 24

Ingredients:

- 1-½ cup unsweetened brown rice cereal
- ¾ cup Old Fashioned oats
- ½ cup hazelnuts or walnuts, coarsely chopped
- ⅓ cup + 2 Tbs. dark chocolate (70% cocoa or greater), chopped into chunks
- 1 cup dates, deglet noor, pureed until smooth
- ½ cup hazelnut butter (can use almond, cashew, or peanut)
- 2 Tbs. liquid Stevia
- 3 tsp. cinnamon

Directions:

(1) In a medium mixing bowl, add cereal, oats, nuts, and cinnamon. Stir until combined well. Set aside.

(2) Melt chocolate in a medium bowl over double boiler. Remove bowl from double boiler. Add dates, butter, and Stevia. Carefully mix with wooden spoon until combined well. If mixture stiffens too much, set bowl over double boiler again as needed.

(3) Add chocolate mixture to cereal mixture. Fold in until thoroughly combined.

(4) Scrape mixture into a 9" x 11" x 2" baking pan, pressing down firmly with your hands and smooth the top.

(5) Cover and refrigerate for 30 minutes to 1 hour, allowing mixture to set.

(6) Cut into 1-½ inch squares and serve. In addition to squares, you can roll mixture into 24 truffle-like balls.

(7) Store remaining squares in refrigerator for up to 5 days.

Sunshine Pumpkin Muffins

Servings: 4

Ingredients:

- 1 cup Old Fashioned oats
- ½ cup amaranth or quinoa flour + ¼ cup coconut flour
- ¼ cup craisins or raisins
- ½ cup unsweetened applesauce + ½ cup canned pure pumpkin
- 2 large egg whites + 1 yolk, beaten lightly
- 3 Tbs. coconut oil
- ½ cup pure unsweetened almond milk
- 1 Tbs. baking powder, double-acting + ½ tsp. baking soda

- 2 tsp. cinnamon + 1-½ tsp. pumpkin pie spice
- ½ tsp. ground nutmeg
- coconut oil cooking spray

Directions:

(1) Preheat oven to 375 degrees Fahrenheit.

(2) Spray muffin pan with coconut oil cooking spray.

(3) In a medium mixing bowl, combine oats and all well ingredients (applesauce, pumpkin, eggs, oil, and almond milk). Add craisins or raisins and mix well.

(4) In a large mixing bowl, combine remaining dry ingredients: baking powder, baking soda, spices, and flours. Mix well. Make a well in the center of the dry ingredients and pour wet ingredients from medium bowl. Mix until all dry ingredients are just moistened. Fill muffin cups to two-thirds full. Bake 15-20 minutes or until lightly browned on top.

(5) Remove from oven when done and let cool in muffin tins for 2-3 minutes. Remove muffins from tin and store in airtight container.

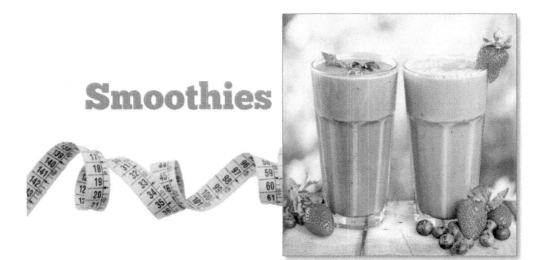

Smoothies

Smoothies are awesome snacks that will provide your body with mega nutrients. Just throw all ingredients into a blender and puree – about 3 minutes. Use your favorite protein powder whether it's made from whey, casein, egg, pea, or hemp. The ForeverYoung.MD SLIM Shake is also a great alternative. Just stick with your protein requirements. If the consistency of your smoothie is too thick, you may add more water. Start with ¼ cup and re-assess before adding more. Each smoothie recipes makes 1 serving. Enjoy!

Avocado Lime Smoothie

- ½ avocado, peeled and pitted
- 1 lime, juice and rind
- 14-28 grams protein powder, vanilla
- 1 Tbs. hemp seeds
- ½ cup almond milk
- ½ Tbs. almond extract
- handful of ice cubes

Berry Boost Smoothie

- ⅓ cup blueberries

- ¾ cup strawberries
- 14-28 grams protein powder, vanilla or chocolate
- 1 Tbs. flaxseed
- 1 Tbs. almonds
- 1 cup cold water
- handful of ice cubes

Chocolate Cranberry Smoothie

- 1 handful of spinach
- 1 cup carrots
- ½ cup frozen cranberries
- ¼ small orange peeled and sliced
- 14-28 grams protein powder, chocolate
- 1 Tbs. almonds
- 1 cup pure unsweetened almond milk
- handful of ice cubes

Cozy Gingerbread Latte Smoothie

- 14-28 grams protein powder, vanilla
- 8 oz. pure unsweetened almond milk
- ½ tsp. vanilla extract
- 1 tsp. molasses
- 1 tsp. ground ginger
- 1 tsp. cinnamon
- ½ tsp. ground cloves
- ¼ tsp. nutmeg
- handful of ice cubes

Go Green Juice Smoothie

- 1 handful of kale, stalks removed
- ½ cup spinach
- 1 cup chopped cucumber

- ⅓ cup frozen raspberries
- ½ cup pineapple, canned in natural juices
- 14-28 grams protein powder, vanilla
- 1 Tbs. chia seeds
- ½ cup light coconut water
- 1 cup pure unsweetened coconut milk
- dash of ginger
- Ice or Water (as desired)

Kale Berry Blend Smoothie

- 1 heaping cup of kale leaves
- ½ cup blackberries
- ½ cup raspberries
- 14-28 grams protein powder, chocolate
- 1 Tbs. chia seeds
- 1 cup cold purified water
- handful of ice cubes

Kale Elixir Smoothie

- 1 heaping cup of kale leaves
- ½ small banana
- 1 date, deglet noor
- 10 oz. pure unsweetened protein powder, vanilla
- ½ tsp. cinnamon
- 1 packet Stevia

Minty Chocolate Shake Smoothie

- 10 fresh mint leaves
- 14-28 grams protein powder
- 2 Tbs. flaxseed
- 8 oz. pure unsweetened almond milk
- handful of ice cubes

Peanut Butter and Chocolate Shake Smoothie

- 1 Tbs. unsweetened cocoa powder
- 14-28 grams protein powder, chocolate
- 2 Tbs. pure peanut butter
- 10 oz. purified water
- ½ tsp. vanilla extract
- 1 packet Stevia
- handful of ice cubes

Pineapple Banana Smoothie

- 1 handful of spinach leaves
- ½ small banana
- ½ cup pineapple chunks
- 14-28 grams protein powder, vanilla
- 2 Tbs. flaxseed
- 1-2 cups purified water
- handful of ice cubes

Water & Tea

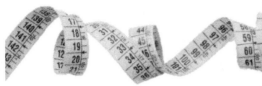
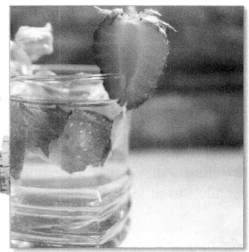

To make your beverages more exciting than the usual water or tea, we are providing you with a few beverage recipes that are extremely beneficial to your body and overall health. Make a pitcher of one or two recipes in the morning and sip for the rest of the day. If you're away from home, fill a large thermos and take with you so that you don't forget to hydrate yourself.

Berry Water

- 1 gallon of purified water
- ½ cup blueberries
- ½ cup raspberries

Directions: Muddle berries in pitcher and add cold water. Place in refrigerator for 30-60 minutes. Stir before serving.

Cucumber Mint Water

- 1 gallon of purified water
- ½ cucumber, sliced
- 4 fresh mint leaves

Directions: Mix all ingredients. Place in refrigerator for 3 hours to chill before serving.

Ginger Tea

- 1 cup hot purified water
- 1 oz. ginger root, peeled

Directions: Add ginger root to hot water for one serving of hot ginger tea. Allow to sit for 8-10 minutes before drinking.

Green Tea

- 2 liters of hot purified water
- 8 organic green tea bags
- 1 organic tangerine, sliced
- 3 fresh mint leaves

Directions: Boil water and pour in pitcher. Add tea bags to steep. After cooling (approximately 30-60 minutes), remove tea bags. Add tangerine and mint leaves. Place in refrigerator for 3 hours before serving.

Herbal Iced Tea

- 2 quarts of purified hot water
- 4 caffeine-free herbal tea bags (chamomile, peach, etc.)
- 8 packets of Stevia (optional)

Directions: Add tea bags to hot water. Let steep for 15-20 minutes. Remove tea bags. Stir in Stevia to sweeten. You may add less or more to your liking. Add ice or place in refrigerator for 3 hours before serving.

Lemonade

- 12 oz. purified water
- 1 lemon, juiced

- 1 packet of Stevia

Directions: Stir lemon and Stevia in water for one serving of refreshing lemonade. Add ice cubes and enjoy!

Mint Tea

- 1 cup hot purified water
- ½ cup fresh mint

Directions: Add mint to hot water and allow infusing for 8-10 minutes before drinking. Makes one serving.

Strawberry Lime Water

- 1 cup of purified water
- 3 organic strawberries
- ½ lime, squeezed

Directions: Cut the tops off the strawberries and cut in halves. Add strawberries and lime to water for one serving of delicious fruity water. Allow 30-60 minutes for fruit and water to infuse before serving.

EPILOGUE

Wise men say the end is just another beginning. This might be the end of the book, but it's only the beginning of a new you forever.

Our sincere hope is that we have introduced you to some of the basic tools you need to get going. Our passion is helping everyone live forever young.

Dropping the fat will get you looking your best, but many of these same principles are intended to get you feeling your best as well. Forever young is a state of mind as much as it is a wellness principle. When you're looking and feeling your physical best, you give your mind, your spirit, and your soul a better opportunity to flourish as well. As you've been reading, our philosophy privileges balance over extremism.

ForeverYoung.MD is about overall healthy dieting choices and complete wellness. Don't get caught up trying to compare yourself with the photos of celebrities on magazine covers. Everyone knows by now that many of these images are digitally enhanced, but what you might not know is that many of these characters also undergo extreme diets and procedures to look the way they do. Those aren't healthy in the long-run. Focus on your own goals and be your own person.

With determination and consistency, you may very well become as fit as some of the models you see on these magazine covers. But you need to be realistic. "Six-pack abs" are not typical even for world-class models. To achieve these photo-perfect results, many of them engage in extreme diet manipulation just prior to the photo shoot. Unless you have a session scheduled with Maxim in the next couple of weeks, these methods are not a good idea for you. A great set of abs is nice, but what's really important is your overall wellbeing. That starts with a balanced approach to dropping the fat.

Your wellness is in your own hands. With the right attitude, resiliency and an open mind, anyone can be forever young. This includes you!

If you would like more information or if you're just looking for a helping hand, please visit our website at www.ForeverYoung.MD.

Lastly, if you have enjoyed our book, please tell us or leave a review at the place you obtained your copy. It's only through feedback that we can enjoy any success getting our message to all those whom it might benefit. Our most earnest efforts and contributions to health mean nothing without your support.

Thank you for reading. Keep thriving to the end!

OTHER BOOKS YOU MAY ENJOY

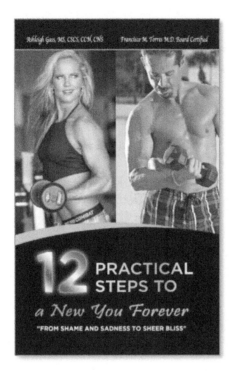

12 Practical Steps to a New You Forever – *From Shame and Sadness to Sheer Bliss*

By Dr. Francisco M. Torres & Ashleigh Gass

12 Practical Steps to a New You Forever Without Arthritis – *Stealing Back Your Life from Pain and Inflammation*

By Dr. Francisco M. Torres & Ashleigh Gass

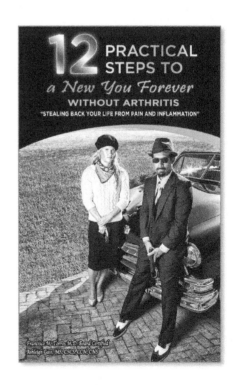

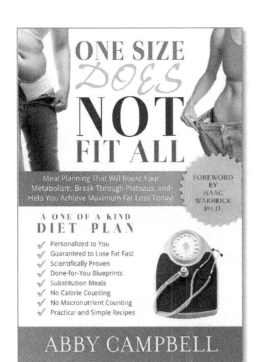

One Size Does NOT Fit All Diet Plan – *Meal Planning That Will Boost Your Metabolism, Break Through Plateaus, and Help You Achieve Maximum Fat Loss Today!*

By Abby Campbell

ENDNOTES

[1] Harvard T.H. Chan School of Public Health. (2015, June 29). *Obesity Has Doubled Since 1980, Major Global Analysis of Risk Factors Revealed.* Retrieved from http://www.hsph.harvard.edu/news/press-releases/worldwide-obesity/.

[2] Yang, L. & Colditz, G. (2015, June 22). Prevalence of Overweight and Obesity in the United States, 2007-2012. *JAMA Internal Medicine.* doi: 10.1001/jamainternmed.2015.2405. Retrieved from http://archinte.jamanetwork.com/article.aspx?articleid=2323411.

[3] Ogden, C., Carroll, M. & Flegal, K. (2008, May). High Body Mass Index for Age Among U.S. Children and Adolescents, 2003-2006. *Journal of American Medical Association, 229(20)*, 2401-2405. doi: 10.1001/jama.229.20.2401. Retrieved from http://jama.ama-assn.org/content/299/20/2401.full.pdf.

[4] United States Department of Agriculture Center for Nutrition Policy and Promotion. (1992, August). *The Food Guide Pyramid, Home and Garden Bulletin Number 252.* Retrieved from http://www.cnpp.usda.gov/Publications/MyPyramid/Original FoodGuidePyramids/FGP/FGPPamphlet.pdf.

[5] Harvard T.H. Chan School of Public Health. (2015, June 29). *An Epidemic of Obesity: U.S. Obesity Trends.* Retrieved from http://www.hsph.harvard.edu/nutritionsource/an-epidemic-of-obesity/.

[6] National Heart, Lung, and Blood Institute. (2015, June 29). *What Are the Signs and Symptoms of Metabolic Syndrome?* Retrieved from http://www.nhlbi.nih.gov/health/health-topics/topics/ms/signs.

[7] Soares, M., Cummings, M., Ping-Delfos, W. (2011, April-June). Energy Metabolism and the Metabolic Syndrome: Does a Lower Basal Metabolic Rate Signal Recovery Following Weight Loss? *Diabetes & Metabolic Syndrome: Clinical Research & Reviews, 5(2)*, 98-101. doi:10.1016/j.dsx.2012.03.003. Retrieved from http://www.sciencedirect.com/science/article/pii/S187140211200032X?np=y.

[8] Berardi, J. & Andrews, R. (2009). The Macronutrients. International Sports Sciences Association. *Nutrition: The Complete Guide* (166-175). Carpinteria, CA: International Sports Sciences Association.

[9] Institute of Medicine of the National Academics (2005). Energy. National Academy of Sciences. *Dietary Reference Intakes for Energy, Carbohydrate, Fiber, Fat, Fatty Acids, Cholesterol, Protein, and Amino Acids* (114). Washington, DC: The National Academies Press.

[10] Blom, W., Lluch, A. & Stafleu, A., et al. (2006, February). Effect of a High-Protein Breakfast on the Postprandial Ghrelin Response. *The American Journal of Clinical*

Nutrition, 83(2), 211-220. Retrieved from
http://www.ajcn.org/content/83/2/211.full.pdf.

[11] Yakar, S., Rosen, C. & Bemer, W., et al. (2002, September 15). Circulating Levels of IGF-1 Directly Regulate Bone Growth and Density. *The Journal of Clinical Investigation, 110(6)*, 771-781. doi: 10.1172/jc115463. Retrieved from http://www.jci.org/articles/view/15463.

[12] Sjogren, K., Leung, K. & Kaplan, W., et al. (2007, April 24). Growth Hormone Regulation of Metabolic Expression in Muscle: A Microarray Study in Hypopituitary Men. *American Journal of Physiology Endocrinology and Metabolism, 293(1)*, E364-E371. doi: 10.1152/ajpendo.00054.2007. Retrieved from http://ajpendo.physiology.org/content/293/1/E364.full.pdf.

[13] Ibid.

[14] Tipton, K., Elliott, T. & Cree, M., et al. (2004, December). Ingestion of Casein and Whey Proteins Result in Muscle Anabolism after Resistance Exercise. *Medicine & Science in Sports & Exercise, 36(12)*, 2073-2081. doi: 10.1249/01/MSS.0000147582.99810.C5. Retrieved from http://www.sportsnutritionworkshop.com/Files/18.SPNT.pdf.

[15] Willett, W. (2010, April 6). Fruits, Vegetables, and Cancer Prevention: Turmoil in the Produce Section. *Journal of the National Cancer Institute, 102(8)*, 510-511. doi: 10.1093/jnci/djq098. Retrieved from http://jnci.oxfordjournals.org/content/102/8/510.full/pdf.

[16] Ness, A. & Powles, J. (1997). Fruit and Vegetables, and Cardiovascular Disease: A Review. *International Journal of Epidemiology, 26(1)*, 1-13. doi: 10.1093/ije/26.1.1. Retrieved from http://ije.oxfordjournals.org/content/26/1/1.full.pdf.

[17] Duncan, K., Bacon, J. & Weinsier, R. (1983, May). The Effects of High and Low Energy Density Diets on Satiety, Energy Intake, and Eating Time of Obese and Nonobese Subjects. *American Journal of Clinical Nutrition, 37(5)*, 763-767. Retrieved from http://www.ajcn.org/content/37/5/763.full.pdf.

[18] Bell, E. & Rolls, B. (2001, June). Energy Density of Foods Affect Energy Intake Across Multiple Levels of Fat Content in Lean and Obese Women. *American Journal of Clinical Nutrition, 73(6)*, 1010-1018. Retrieved from http://www.ajcn.org/content/73/6/1010.full.pdf.

[19] Berardi, J. & Andrews, R. (2009). The Macronutrients. International Sports Sciences Association. Nutrition: The Complete Guide (149-156). Carpinteria, CA: International Sports Sciences Association.

[20] Slowik, G. (2012, March 22). Fiber: Its Importance In Your Diet. Retrieved from http://ehealthmd.com/content/what-fiber.

[21] Berardi, J. & Andrews, R. (2009). The Macronutrients. International Sports Sciences Association. Nutrition: The Complete Guide (146-156). Carpinteria, CA: International Sports Sciences Association.

[22] National Institutes of Health Office of Dietary Supplements. (2015, June 30). *Vitamin C.* Retrieved from http://ods.od.nih.gov/factsheets/VitaminC-HealthProfessional/.

[23] Perlmutter, D. (2013). Grain Brain: The Surprising Truth About Wheat, Carbs, and Sugar – Your Brain's Silent Killers. New York, New York: Little, Brown and Company.

[24] Liese, A., Roach, A. & Sparks, K., et al. (2003, November). Whole-Grain Intake and Insulin Sensitivity: The Insulin Resistance Atherosclerosis Study. *The American Journal of Clinical Nutrition, 78(5)*, 965-971. Retrieved from http://www.ajcn.org/content/78/5/965.full.pdf.

[25] Meyer, K., Kushi, L. & Jacobs, D., et al. (2000, April). Carbohydrates, Dietary Fiber, and Incident Type 2 Diabetes in Older Women. *The American Journal of Clinical Nutrition, 71(4)*, 921-930. Retrieved from http://www.ajcn.org/content/71/4/921.full.pdf.

[26] Hu, F. (2010, April 21). Are Refined Carbohydrates Worse Than Saturated Fats? *The American Journal of Clinical Nutrition, 91(6)*, 1541-1542. Retrieved from http://www.ajcn.org/content/91/6/1541.full.pdf.

[27] Breen, L., Philp, A. & Witard, O., et al. (2011, July 11). The Influence of True Carbohydrate-Protein Co-Ingestion Following Endurance Exercise of Myofibrillar and Mitochondrial Protein Synthesis. *The Journal of Physiology, 589*, 4011-4025. doi: 10.113/jphysiol.2011.211888. Retrieved from http://jp.physoc.org/content/589/16/4011.full.pdf.

[28] Ivy, J., Lee, M. & Brozinick, J., et al. (1988). Muscle Glycogen Storage After Different Amounts of Carbohydrate Ingestion. *Journal of Applied Physiology, 65(5)*, 2018-2023. Retrieved from http://www.deepdyve.com/lp/the-american-physiological-society/muscle-glycogen-storage-after-different-amounts-of-carbohydrate-153asrxeem.

[29] Berardi, J. & Andrews, R. (2009). The Macronutrients. International Sports Sciences Association. Nutrition: The Complete Guide (157-165). Carpinteria, CA: International Sports Sciences Association.

[30] Christen, W., Schaumber, D. & Glynn, R., et al. (2011, June). Dietary w-3 Fatty Acid and Fish Intake and Incident Age-Related Macular Degeneration in Women. *JAMA Ophthalmology, 129(7)*, 921-929. doi 10.1001/archophthalmol.2011.34. Retrieved from http://archopht.jamanetwork.com/article.aspx?articleid=1106372.

[31] Mozaffarian, D., Katan, M. & Ascherio, A., et al. (2006, April 13). Trans Fatty Acids and Cardiovascular Disease. *The New England Journal of Medicine, 354*, 1601-1613.

[32] Grimm, M., Rothhaar, T. & Grosgen, S., et al. (2011, June 29). Trans Fatty Acids Enhance Amyloidogenic Processing of Alzheimer Amyloid Precursor Protein (APP). *The Journal of Nutritional Biochemistry*. doi: 10.1016/jnutbio.2011.06.015.

[33] Hu, J., Vecchia, C. & de Groh, M., et al. (2011, November). Dietary Trans Fatty Acids and Cancer Risk. *European Journal of Cancer Prevention, 20(6)*, 530-538. doi: 10.1097/CEJ/0b013e328348fbfb.

[34] Freund, Y., Vedin, I. & Cederholm, T., et al. (2014, January 11). Transfer of Omega-3 Fatty Acids Across the Blood-Brain Barrier After Dietary Supplementation with a Docosahexaenoic Acid-Rich Omega-3 Fatty Acid Preparation in Patients with Alzheimer's Disease: The OmegaAD Study. *Journal of Internal Medicine, 275(4)*, 428-436. doi: 10.1111/joim.12166. Retrieved from http://onlinelibrary.wiley.com/doi/10.1111/joim.12166/full.

[35] Gonzalez-Periz, A., Horrillo, R. & Ferre, N., et al. (2009, February 11). Obesity-Induced Insulin Resistance and Hepatic Steatosis are Alleviated by Omega-3 Fatty Acids: A Role for Resolvins and Protectins. *The FASEB Journal, 23(6)*, 1946-1957. doi: 10.1096/fj.08-125674. Retrieved from http://www.fasebj.org/content/23/6/1946.full.pdf.

[36] Coreet, C., Delarue, J. & Ritz. P., et al. (1997, July 22). Effect of Dietary Fish Oil on Body Fat Mass and Basal Fat Oxidation in Healthy Adults. *International Journal of Obesity, 21*, 632-643. doi: 10.1038/sj.ijo.0800451. Retrieved from http://www.nature.com/ijo/journal/v21/n8/pdf/0800451a.pdf.

[37] Musumeci, G., Frovato, F & Pichier, K. (2013, December). Extra-Virgin Olive Oil Diet and Mild Physical Activity Prevent Cartilage Degeneration in an Osteoarthritis Model: An In Vivo and In Vitro Study on Lubricin Expression. *The Journal of Nutritional Biochemistry, 24(12)*, 2064-2075. Retrieved from http://www.ncbi.nlm.nih.gov/pubmed/24369033.

[38] St-Onge, M. & Bosarge, A. (2008, March). Weight-Loss Diet that Includes Consumption of Medium-Chain Triacylglycerol Oil Leads to a Greater Rate of Weight and Fat Mass Loss than Does Olive Oil. *The American Journal of Clinical Nutrition, 87(3)*, 621-626. Retrieved from http://ajcn.nutrition.org/content/87/3/621.long.

[39] Avena, N., Rada, P. & Hoebel, B. (2008). Evidence for Sugar Addiction: Behavior and Neurochemical Effects of Intermittent, Excessive Sugar Intake. *Neuroscience & Biobehavioral Reviews, 32(1)*, 20-39. Retrieved from http://www.ncbi.nlm.nih.gov/pmc/articles/PMC2235907/pdf/nihms36189.pdf.

[40] Berardi, J. & Andrews, R. (2009). Water and Fluid Balance. International Sports Sciences Association. Nutrition: The Complete Guide (207-224). Carpinteria, CA: International Sports Sciences Association.

[41] Dennis, E., Dengo, A. & Comber, D., et al. (2010, February). Water Consumption Increases Weight Loss During a Hypocaloric Diet Intervention in Middle-Aged and

Older Adults. *Obesity, 18(2)*, 300-307. doi: 10.1038/oby.2009.235. Retrieved from http://www.ipwr.org/documents/WaterWeightLoss.Obesity.2009.pdf.

[42] Han, C. (2011, November). Studies on Tea and Health. *Wei Sheng Yan Jiu, 40(6)*, 802-805.

[43] Serafini, M., Del Rio, D. & Yao, D., et al. (2011). Health Benefits of Tea. Benzie, I.F.F. & Wachtel-Galor, S. *Herbal Medicine: Biomolecular and Clinical Aspects* (239-262). Boca Raton, FL: Taylor and Francis Group, LLC.

[44] Auvichayapat, P. Prapochanung, M. & Tunkamnerdthai, O., et al. (2008, February 27). Effectiveness of Green Tea on Weight Reduction in Obese Thais: A Randomized, Controlled Trial. *Physiology & Behavioral 93(3)*, 486-491. doi: 10.1016/j.physbeh2007.10.009.

[45] English, K. & Paddon-Jone, D. (2010, January). Protecting Muscle Mass and Function in Older Adults During Bed Rest. *Current Opinion in Clinical Nutrition and Metabolic Care, 13(1)*, 34-39. doi: 10.1097/MCO.0b013e328333aa66. Retrieved from http://www.ncbi.nlm.nih.gov/pmc/articles/PMC3276215/pdf/nihms-181019.pdf.

[46] Bishop-Bailey, D. (2013, November). Mechanisms Governing the Health and Performance Benefits of Exercise. *British Journal of Pharmacology, 170(6)*, 1153-1166. doi: 10.1111/bph.123999. Retrieved from http://www.ncbi.nlm.nih.gov/pmc/articles/PMC2235907/pdf/nihms36189.pdf.

[47] Ibid.

[48] Ibid.

[49] Ibid.

[50] Ibid.

[51] American Heart Association®. (2015, August 17). *American Heart Association Recommendations for Physical Activity in Adults.* Retrieved from http://www.heart.org/HEARTORG/GettingHealthy/PhysicalActivity/FitnessBasics/American-Heart-Association-Recommendations-for-Physical-Activity-in-Adults_UCM_307976_Article.jsp.

[52] Francis, M. & Pennebaker, J. (1992, March-April). Putting Stress Into Words: The Impact of Writing on Physiological, Absentee, and Self-Reported Emotional Wellbeing Measures. *American Journal of Health Promotion, 6(4)*, 280-287. Retrieved from http://www.ncbi.nlm.nih.gov/pubmed/10146806.

[53] West, J., Otte, C. & Geher, K., et al. (2004, October). Effects of Hatha Yoga and African Dance on Perceived Stress, Affect, and Salivary Cortisol. *Annals of Behavioral Medicine, 28(2)*, 114-118. Retrieved from http://link.springer.com/article/10.1207%2Fs15324796abm2802_6.

[54] Sanchez, B., Gonzalez-Rodriguez, I. & Arboleva, S., et al. (2015, February 22). The Effects of Bifidobacterium Breve on Immune Mediators and Proteome of HT29 Cells Monolayers. *BioMed Research International.* doi:10.1155/2015/479140. Retrieved from http://www.ncbi.nlm.nih.gov/pmc/articles/PMC4352474/.

[55] Soltan-Dallal, M., Mojarrad,M. & Baghbani, F., et al. (2015, March). Effects of Probiotic Lactobacillus Acidophilus and Lactobacillus Casei on Colorectoral Tumor Cells Activity (CaCO-2). *Archives of Iranian Medicine, 18(3)*, 167-172. doi: 0151803/AIM.006. Retrieved from http://www.ams.ac.ir/AIM/NEWPUB/15/18/3/006.pdf.

[56] Deepak, V., Pandian, S. & Sivasubramaniam, S., et al. (2015, April 1). Optimization of Anticancer Exopolysaccharide Production from Probiotic Lactobacillus Acidophilus by Response Surface Methodology. *Preparative Biochemistry and Biotechnology.* doi: 10.1080/10826068.2015.1031386. Retrieved from http://www.tandfonline.com/doi/abs/10.1080/10826068.2015.1031386?url_ver=Z39.88-2003&rfr_id=ori:rid:crossref.org&rfr_dat=cr_pub%3dpubmed.

[57] Saez-Lara, M., Gomez-Llorente, C. & Plaza-Diaz, J., et al. (2015, February 22). The Role of Probiotic Lactic Acid Bacteria and Bifidobacteria in the Prevention and Treatment of Inflammatory Bowel Disease and Other Related Diseases: A Systematic Review of Randomized Human Clinical Trials. *BioMed Research International.* doi: 10.1155/2015/505878. Retrieved from http://www.ncbi.nlm.nih.gov/pmc/articles/PMC4352483/.

[58] Wasilewski, A., Zielinska, M. & Storr, M., et al. (2015, March 27). Beneficial Effects of Probiotics, Synbiotics, and Psychobiotics in Inflammatory Bowel Disease. *Inflammatory Bowel Disease.* doi: 10.1097/MIB.0000000000000364. Retrieved from http://www.tandfonline.com/doi/abs/10.1080/10826068.2015.1031386?url_ver=Z39.88-2003&rfr_id=ori:rid:crossref.org&rfr_dat=cr_pub%3dpubmed.

[59] Choi, C., Kwon, J. & Kim, S. (2015, March 25). Efficacy of Combination Therapy with Probiotics and Mosapride in Patients with IBS without Diarrhea: A Randomized, Double-Blind, Placebo-Controlled Multicenter, Phase II Trial. *Neurogastroenterology & Motility.* doi: 10.1111.nmo.12544. Retrieved from http://onlinelibrary.wiley.com/doi/10.1111/nmo.12544/abstract;jsessionid=14DDCC0E273A370B0D81D47A3C7E29DC.f01t03.

[60] Anandharaj, M., Sivansankari, B. & Santhanakaruppu, R., et al. (2015, April 1). Determining the Probiotic Potential of Cholesterol-Reducing Lactobacillus and Weissella Strains Isolated for Gherkins (Fermented Cucumber) and South Indian Ferment Koozh. *Research in Microbiology.* doi: 10.1016/j.resmic.2015.03.002. Retrieved from http://www.ncbi.nlm.nih.gov/pubmed/25839996.

[61] Swain, M., Anandharai, M. & Ray, R., et al. (2014). Fermented Fruits and Vegetables of Asia: A Potential Source of Probiotics. *Biotechnology Research International.* doi: 10.1155/2014/250424. Retrieved from http://www.ncbi.nlm.nih.gov/pmc/articles/PMC4058509/.

[62] Park, K., Jeong, J. & Lee, Y., et al. (2014, January). Health Benefits of Kimchi (Korean Fermented Vegetables) as a Probiotic Food. *Journal of Medicinal Food, 17(1)*, 6-20. doi: 10.1089/jmf.2013.3083. Retrieved from http://online.liebertpub.com/doi/abs/10.1089/jmf.2013.3083.

[63] Nguyen, N., Dong, N. & Nguyen, H., et al. (2015, February 24). Lactic Acid Bacteria: Promising Supplements for Enhancing the Biological Activities of Kombucha. *Springerplus, 4(91)*. doi: 10.1186/s40064-015-0872-3. Retrieved from http://www.ncbi.nlm.nih.gov/pmc/articles/PMC4348356/.

[64] Banerjee, D., Hassarajani, S. & Maity, B., et al. (2010, December). Comparative Healing Property of Kombucha Tea and Black Tea Against Indomethacin-Induced Gastric Ulceration in Mice: Possible Mechanism of Action. *Food & Function, 3*, 284-293. doi: 10.1039/C0FO00025F. Retrieved from http://pubs.rsc.org/en/Content/ArticleLanding/2010/FO/c0fo00025f.

[65] Yu, J., Gao, W. & Qing, M., et al. (2012). Identification and Characterization of Lactic Acid Bacteria Isolated from Traditional Pickles in Sichuan, China. *The Journal of General and Applied Microbiology, 58(3)*, 163-172. doi: 10.2323/jgam.58.163. Retrieved from https://www.jstage.jst.go.jp/article/jgam/58/3/58_163/_pdf.

[66] Raak, C., Ostermann, T. & Boehm, K., et al. (2014, November). Regular Consumption of Sauerkraut and Its Effect on Human Health: A Bibliometric Analysis. *Global Advances in Health and Medicine, 3 (6)*, 12-18. doi: 10.7453/gahmj.2014.038. Retrieved from http://www.ncbi.nlm.nih.gov/pubmed/25568828.

[67] Consumer Reports Food Safety and Sustainability Center. (2015, April). From Crop to Table Pesticide Use in Produce. Retrieved from http://www.consumerreports.org/content/dam/cro/magazine-articles/2015/May/Consumer%20Reports_From%20Crop%20to%20Table%20Report_March%202015.pdf.

[68] United States Department of Agriculture. (2013, July). Organic Livestock Requirements. USDA National Organic Progra | Agricultural Marketing. Retrieved from http://www.ams.usda.gov/AMSv1.0/getfile?dDocName=STELPRDC5102526.

Made in the USA
Columbia, SC
04 February 2021